1998 January

$26.63

Featuring
50 Powerful Herbal Cures

1998

NATURAL HEALING REMEDIES

How to Guard Your Health,
Boost Your Immunity,
and Banish Fatigue

Edited by Doug Dollemore, **PREVENTION** Health Books™

Rodale Press, Inc.
Emmaus, Pennsylvania

Notice

This book is intended as a reference volume only, not as a medical manual. The information given here is designed to help you make informed decisions about your health. It is not intended as a substitute for any treatment that may have been prescribed by your doctor. If you suspect that you have a medical problem, we urge you to seek competent medical help.

ISBN 0–87596–534–2 hardcover
ISBN 0–87596–538–5 paperback

Distributed in the book trade by St. Martin's Press

2 4 6 8 10 9 7 5 3 1 hardcover
2 4 6 8 10 9 7 5 3 1 paperback

—— OUR PURPOSE ——

"We inspire and enable people to improve their lives and the world around them."

Natural Healing Remedies Editorial Staff

Senior Managing Editor: Edward Claflin
Editor: Doug Dollemore
Managing Editor, *Prevention* Magazine: Marty Munson
Writer: Alisa Bauman
Assistant Research Manager: Anita C. Small
Lead Researcher: Jennifer Barefoot
Editorial Researchers: Carol J. Gilmore, Deborah J. Pedron
Senior Copy Editor: Kathy D. Everleth
Copy Editors: Kathy A. Cressman, Linda Mooney
Cover and Book Designer: Kristen Morgan Downey
Interior Photographer: Mitch Mandel
Layout Designer: Faith Hague
Manufacturing Coordinator: Patrick T. Smith
Office Manager: Roberta Mulliner
Office Staff: Julie Kehs, Bernadette Sauerwine

Rodale Health and Fitness Books

Vice-President and Editorial Director: Debora T. Yost
Executive Editor: Neil Wertheimer
Design and Production Director: Michael Ward
Research Manager: Ann Gossy Yermish
Copy Manager: Lisa D. Andruscavage
Book Manufacturing Director: Helen Clogston

Contents

Part 1
Natural Healing: The Herbal Way
The Best and Brightest Possibilities for Herbal Remedies

Part 2
The Herbal Pharmacy
Natural Prescriptions for Healing

Part 3
Nature's Best Healers
Quick Access to Pill-Free Remedies

115 Aches and Pains

There should be a mirror up there on the painkiller shelves because you may already be holding the real key to pain relief—in your mind.

123 Allergies

Usually, your immune system wages battle against potentially harmful invaders. But if you're one of the many Americans with allergies, your immune system becomes just a little too efficient, and that's when trouble can ensue.

128 Arthritis

If you thought the last word on arthritis was, "Pop painkillers and suffer," you haven't been talking to the right sources. New research brings hope that what you eat can ease your pain.

Contents

Part 4
Timely Paths to Natural Health
An Overview of the Best New Programs, Plans, and Ideas in Natural Healing

Introduction

Back in the days when James A. Duke, Ph.D., went trekking through the jungles of Panama in search of wild botanicals for the U.S. Department of Agriculture, he had an opportunity to try out some of the local food. Unfortunately, food poisoning set in, and Dr. Duke became so weak that he was unable to stand up, let alone work.

Dr. Duke visited some local M.D.'s, but he found that U.S.-style pharmaceutical medicines did little good. Finally, he visited a "more herbally inclined" Panamanian doctor, who gave him powdered carob, used locally to help cure food poisoning.

Dr. Duke's condition improved immediately. And 30 years later, when he read a study in a medical journal about the curative effects of carob powder, Dr. Duke could give firsthand testimony to its healing powers.

Of course, many of us aren't quite as adventurous as Dr. Duke—or the many other authorities on natural healing who are featured in this book. The fact is, many of us are born skeptics, and we harbor some suspicion—or queasiness—about things that are new, especially when we're offered them for ingestion. But we can be open-minded enough to appreciate that others have gone ahead and explored—and to learn from their daring. In the spirit of these pioneers, maybe we'll also be open-minded enough to try new things and learn to appreciate them.

As we become increasingly aware that modern medicine is not only fallible but sometimes downright risky, more and more people are dabbling with a wondrous array of natural cures. And much to their surprise and delight, people are finding that these safe, effective, and easy-to-use remedies are curing what ails them. Intrigued, they ask, "Got any more?"

Our answer is a resounding yes. In this edition of *Natural Healing Remedies*, we focus on one of the oldest natural healers: Herbs. In part 1, Natural Healing: The Herbal Way, some of the nation's top herbal experts, including Dr. Duke, discuss the basics that you'll need to grow, gather, store, and use herbs safely. In part 2, The Herbal Pharmacy, our panel of experts share their accumulated wisdom about getting the most from 50 of the world's most potent medicinal herbs. In Nature's Best Healers—

part 3—we take an in-depth look at 18 common ailments and the dozens of natural treatments, including herbs, food, and exercise, that can prevent or cure them. Finally, in part 4, Timely Paths to Natural Health, world-renowned alternative-medicine practitioners, including Andrew Weil, M.D., and Herbert Benson, M.D., show you ways that you can painlessly weave these herbal and other natural-healing techniques into your everyday life.

If you haven't tried herbs or other natural remedies before, you've been missing more than a dose of powdered carob. Many of these remedies not only perk you up and make you feel better in the short term but also offer you the opportunity of substantial long-term gains in health—improvements that can make you feel younger, help prevent serious problems like diabetes and heart disease, and even help you live a longer, more energetic life.

So here's a full plate. Try a sampling or two. Even if some of these remedies are a novelty to you, we suspect that when you start to follow the natural healers who are leading the way, you'll begin to find out how much of your well-being really is in your own hands. And your willingness to explore may unlock the doors to a healthier future.

Doug Dollemore
Prevention Health Books

part 1

Natural Healing: The Herbal Way

The Best and Brightest

Possibilities

for Herbal Remedies

Why Use Herbs?

*Herbs, the "roots" of modern medicine, have healing
powers that many physicians and consumers are just
beginning to explore and exploit.*

It's amazing where you can find herbal treatments these days.

A 39-year-old woman who had just had surgery to remove a cancerous breast tumor met with radiation oncologist Jerold Green, M.D., at California Pacific Medical Center's gleaming, high-tech radiation oncology unit in San Francisco. Dr. Green explained how he planned to treat her breast with x-rays to kill any cancer cells that the surgery had missed. He also explained that unless she took precautions, the treatments would cause a radiation burn on her breast resembling a bad sunburn. His recommendation was aloe vera gel, extracted from an herb that has been used to treat burns for more than 3,000 years. "Buy it at your pharmacy or at any health food store," Dr. Green says. "Just rub it on your breast before and after each treatment."

A decade ago, most physicians scoffed at medicinal herbs. Some still do. But today, medical journals are publishing more herb research than ever. Consumers, who are fascinated by herbal medicine, continually ask their doctors about it. And the threat of plant extinctions has spurred new scientific interest in the healing power of botanicals. As a result, many mainstream doctors are now incorporating herbs into their practices, says Michael Castleman, author of *Nature's Cures*.

Harvey Komet, M.D., a San Antonio ear, nose, and throat specialist, for example, prescribes gingko to patients with chronic tinnitus, or ringing in their ears—a condition that is notoriously difficult to treat. "I've gotten good results with gingko," he says.

Anne Simon, M.D., assistant clinical professor of family and community medicine at the University of California's San Francisco Medical Center and author of *Before You Call the Doctor*, suggests echinacea for colds and flu. "Studies show that it has an antiviral effect," she explains. "I use it myself."

And gynecologist Dorothy Barbo, M.D., director of the Center for Women's Health at the University of New Mexico in Albuquerque, recommends cranberry juice to prevent bladder infections and as a complement to antibiotics used to treat the infections. "Cranberry juice seems to inhibit bacterial growth," she explains.

Other physicians now tout feverfew to prevent migraine headaches, garlic to control cholesterol levels, saw palmetto to treat prostate enlargement, willow bark to prevent heart attack, and ginger to relieve nausea. Medicine is moving forward into its herbal past as consumers and doctors alike rediscover the "roots" of healing—not to mention its leaves, stems, and flowers.

Herbal Medicine: Ancient and Thoroughly Modern

The botanical roots of modern medicine are everywhere—if you know where to look. Five thousand years ago, Chinese physicians discovered that a tea made from the ma huang plant, Chinese ephedra, relieved asthma and chest congestion.

Today, few people who take over-the-counter decongestants have any idea that they're taking a chemical modeled after a constituent of ephedra. "One chemical in Chinese ephedra is the decongestant pseudoephedrine," explains Varro E. Tyler, Ph.D., Sc.D., former professor of pharmacognosy at Purdue University in West Lafayette, Indiana, and author of *The New Honest Herbal* and *Herbs of Choice*. Pharmaceutical companies now synthesize pseudoephedrine as the decongestant in Actifed, Allerest, Contac, Tylenol Cold and Flu, Nyquil, Formula 44, and other cold formulas and allergy products. One brand—Sudafed—even takes its name from pseudoephedrine.

Ancient India's traditional Ayurvedic medicine dates back 4,500 years to the ancient Hindu text, the *Rig-Veda,* which mentions 67 medicinal herbs, including senna to treat constipation and cinnamon for stomach upsets. These herbs are still used medicinally.

"Senna contains anthraquinone glycosides, chemicals that have powerful laxative action," says James A. Duke, Ph.D., a retired U.S. Department of Agriculture botanist and author of *The Green Pharmacy*. Senna is an ingredient in many commercial laxatives, including Gentlax, Senokot, Fletcher's Castoria, and Innerclean herbal laxative.

"Cinnamon helps relieve stomach distress because its oil has antimicrobial properties," says Daniel Mowrey, Ph.D., director of the American Phytotherapy (plant medicine) Research Laboratory in Salt Lake City and author of *The Scientific Validation of Herbal Medicine.*

Today, we have better treatments for intestinal infections, but cinnamon has been incorporated into several toothpastes, in part because it tastes good but also because its antibiotic action helps kill the bacteria that cause tooth decay and gum disease, says Castleman.

And so it goes. Untold numbers of herbs used in healing during ancient times are still in use today, many of them incorporated into common over-the-counter and prescription medications. And researchers are continually finding new uses for medicinal plants.

Acceptance Grows

These days, ever-increasing numbers of people are returning to herbs—or learning about them for the first time. Herbal teas line supermarket shelves, and most health food stores do a brisk business in medicinal herb teas and tinctures (the liquid form of the herb plus alcohol).

Recently, a woman who was about to begin chemotherapy following surgery to remove a malignant colon tumor met with her oncologist, Barry Rosenbloom, M.D., at Cedars-Sinai Medical Center in Los Angeles. After describing his state-of-the-art, three-drug chemotherapy program, Dr. Rosenbloom mentioned the treatment's major side effect: nausea. But he assured the woman that he could prescribe medication to treat it. "Oh, no," the woman thought, "not another drug."

Anticipating nausea from chemotherapy, the woman had already decided that she wanted to try a friend's herbal treatment of ginger tea. She expected her oncologist to oppose the idea, so her friend armed her with information about research on ginger. (A scientific study showed that ginger relieves the nausea of motion sickness better than a standard pharmaceutical treatment, Dramamine.) The woman told Dr. Rosenbloom that instead of the anti-nausea drug, she'd really rather use ginger. Then she braced herself for an argument.

"Ginger?" Dr. Rosenbloom said. "Sure, why not? It's very good for nausea. Drink ginger ale or grind up the fresh root and make tea. You know, ginger has been used to treat nausea for thousands of years."

Stuck in Regulatory Limbo

If herbs are so great, why aren't they more widely known and used? To claim that any herb or pharmaceutical has medicinal value, it must be either a traditional medicine specifically exempted from current Food and Drug Administration (FDA) regulations, or it must win FDA approval by passing a series of rigorous scientific tests. In the early 1960s, when current FDA rules were drafted, herbal medicine was nowhere near as popular as it is today, so only a few herbs were grandfathered in. One was mint, which contains menthol, an approved treatment for nasal and chest congestion. But the vast majority of herbs were not exempted, Castleman says. They were ignored.

The FDA approval process costs a fortune—more than $100 million per drug. Large pharmaceutical companies have these vast sums and are willing to invest them because new drugs can be patented and sold, often at high prices, to recoup development and approval costs. "But no one is going to put up that kind of money to prove to the FDA that garlic lowers cholesterol," says Mark Blumenthal, executive director of the American Botanical Council in Austin, Texas, and editor of the medicinal herb research journal, *Herbal Gram*. "Many studies show that it does, but the FDA can't grant anyone exclusive rights to garlic, so there's no way to recoup the approval costs," he says. "The same goes for literally hundreds of other herbal medicines. You can't patent plants, so under current FDA regulations, there's no incentive to get them approved for medicinal use."

As a result, most medicinal herbs exist in regulatory limbo. They are sold as foods, not as medicines. Blumenthal and other herb advocates are working to change this situation, but in an odd way, it reflects herbal medicine's place in the natural world. The cultures that gave us medicinal herbs drew no distinction between foods and drugs. Traditional healers around the world have always said, "Let your food be your medicine."

Healing, Not Just Relieving

Herbal medicine works best when practiced holistically—that is, with an intent to heal the entire body and get at the sources of physical and emotional imbalance, instead of just treating the symptoms. For example, if you tend to get headaches, you can use herbs not only to ease the pain but also to eliminate the underlying condition causing the pain. This would eventually restore health and balance so that you no longer get headaches. That is real healing. To achieve this kind of result, a new look at health and healing is required. You must consider not only what you may be taking as medicine—both herbs and drugs—but also your diet, your lifestyle, your mental attitude, and the role that these factors play in keeping you healthy or contributing to disease.

Both traditional herbalists and modern herbal researchers believe that herbs, when properly used, encourage the body to heal itself. Herbal researcher Hildebert Wagner, Ph.D., of the Institute of Munich specializes in studying herbs that improve immunity. He describes herbs as inherently health-promoting rather than disease-killing. "With herbal remedies it is not so much a case of totally blocking a reaction in the organism, as, for example, with cortisone or chemotherapy. Herbal preparations serve very often to regulate and stimulate the organism to promote self-healing tendencies."

The actions of many herbs can be compared with a tap on the shoulder, whereas the effects of drugs can be compared with a kick in the pants. In some cases the body will take longer to heal itself with herbs than it would with quick-acting drugs, but the long-term result is much deeper healing. For many people it's well worth the wait, says Kathi Keville, director of the American Herb Association and author of *Herbs for Health and Healing*.

Herbalism also emphasizes preventive medicine. The point of many herbal treatments is to keep you from getting sick in the first place. We could all take a hint from the traditions of ancient China, where doctors were paid only when they kept their patients well.

Nature Is Often the Best Healer

Most medicinal herbs contain many natural compounds that play off one another, producing a wide variety of results. Even medical science does not always understand how the compounds work together, or even exactly what they all are. As botanist Walter Lewis, Ph.D., and microbiologist Memory Elvin-Lewis, Ph.D., put it in their book *Medical Botany*, "Nature is still mankind's greatest chemist, and many compounds that remain undiscovered in plants are beyond the imagination of even our best scientists."

Some herbs that regulate the body almost seem to have an inner intelligence, with the ability to perform many different functions, depending on what the individual needs, Keville says. For example, ginger can raise or lower blood pressure, depending on what needs to happen to bring an individual's blood pressure to a healthy level. And tonic herbs do more than clear up immediate, acute symptoms; they have the more general effect of renewing strength and vitality. Marsh mallow, for instance, strengthens your digestive system and improves the functioning of your immune system while relieving your stomach distress, says Keville.

Although 80 percent of pharmaceutical drugs are based on herbs, these drugs are generally based not on the whole herb but on one "active ingredient" derived from a plant. Modern medicine has become captivated by what it calls a magic bullet—a single substance that zeros in and destroys a germ or relieves a symptom, Keville says. Whenever possible, the chemical structure of the active component found in an herb is duplicated in the laboratory and produced synthetically. This enables a drug company to produce formulas of consistent quality and strength and avoid the hassle and expense of collecting plants in the wild. (Not incidentally, it also enables them to patent the remedy and charge more money for it, Keville says.)

These magic-bullet drugs have several problems. First, they treat only specific problems. Dr. Duke points out that "the solitary synthetic bullet offers no alternatives if the doctor has misdiagnosed the ailment or if one or more ailments require more than one compound." Herbs, on the other hand, can cover many bases at once.

Magic bullets don't give the body a chance to find its own solution. Dr. Duke theorizes that our bodies take fuller advantage than we realize of the complex chemistry in medicinal herbs. He believes that each herb contains hundreds of active compounds, many of which act synergistically. That means that all these compounds somehow combine to produce a greater effect than each has alone, and that the body extracts the compounds it needs and discards the others. One possible reason that scientific studies sometimes fail to confirm an herb's traditional use in healing is that the studies often focus only on the isolated compound, not on the whole plant.

Years ago, researchers extracted an active compound called silymarin from the herb milk thistle and turned it into a pharmaceutical drug to treat liver damage. Only later did German scientists discover yet another compound in milk thistle—betaine hydrocholoride—that may be equally important.

The popular immunity-enhancing herb echinacea has a similar story. For years, complex carbohydrates from echinacea were thought to be its sole active ingredient and were extracted to produce a drug. But then a team of German researchers headed by Dr. Wagner discovered that echinacea contains other compounds that enhance immunity.

In the case of the sedative herb valerian, medical researchers found that two compounds—valeric acid and essential oils—caused its calming effects, but for some time they remained unaware of still a third set of highly sedative compounds called valepotriates. And gingko, which is used to boost brain functions and circulation, has been found to be more effective when used in its whole form instead of when only its isolated active compounds are used.

Sidestepping Side Effects

Unfortunately, even when a potent magic-bullet drug is right on the mark when it comes to resolving a certain problem, it often creates side effects—new problems. "Scarcely a month goes by without a drug being removed from the market because it is harmful," says Dr. Wagner. "This has helped to let the pendulum swing back and has brought a renewed consideration for our old treasures of experience with herbs."

The FDA receives more than 10,000 reports of side effects from newly approved drugs every year, according to the Center for Drug Evaluation and Research in Rockville, Maryland. This is especially sobering when you consider that about 25 percent of these side effects resulted in someone being hospitalized or dying. And that's only the tip of the iceberg. National surveys indicate that only about 5 percent of serious side effects from drugs are even reported to the center. The Environmental Protection Agency reports that 125,000 Americans die each year because they take their prescribed medicines incorrectly. In fact, some studies indicate that as many as half of all pharmaceuticals are not being taken correctly.

The herbs suggested in this book, however, produce few side effects, and many of them contain protective compounds that keep their potency in check. The herb meadowsweet, which contains natural aspirin (salicylic acid), is a perfect example. As you probably know, a big problem with taking chemical aspirin is that it can injure the stomach lining and even cause bleeding. Meadowsweet functions like aspirin to ease the pain and inflammation of rheumatism and headaches, but it also contains astringent tannins and soothing mucilage, compounds that researchers believe buffer salicylic acid's adverse side effects.

Dr. Duke speculates that the effectiveness of herbs and their less toxic effects on our bodies may be due to our long history of using medicinal plants. "We have adapted ways to be more responsive to herbs," he says. "In many cases your body, through evolution, has been exposed to these natural compounds. Perhaps it has evolved protective mechanisms against their negative effects while embracing their positive effects."

Herbal Cures Are Ecological and Ethical

Another plus for herbal medicine is that it is environmentally sound. One person who has considered the relationship between environmental pollution and drugs is English herbalist David Hoffmann. Author of a number of herb books, including *The Holistic Herbal, Successful Stress Control*, and *The Complete Illustrated Holistic Herbal*, Hoffmann's major issue when he ran for Parliament in England was global ecology. He focused on what happens when you regularly take a common drug used to treat stomach ulcers and gastritis: "You become very involved in an ecological cycle that involves all the pollution produced in the factories that prepare the drug. It just happens that in this process of healing our ulcers, we buy into killing fish—into environmental destruction—and we legitimize the destruction of laboratory animals. Is that healing? I suggest that it is not."

Hoffmann also points out that the pharmaceutical industry is one of the biggest practitioners of vivisection (operating on a living animal for research purposes). The research and development of new drugs generally involves killing thousands of laboratory animals. The resulting drugs are then tested on more animals before being declared safe for humans. "You can sip herbal tea without worrying that a rat or a guinea pig had to die to enable you to do so," he says.

Instead of contributing to destroying the environment, herbs bring us closer to it. Herbalist and acupuncturist Michael Tierra, author of *Planetary Herbology*, believes that herbs can make us more conscious of our place among all of Earth's living things. "The path of the herbalist is one that can offer a vital link to the natural and interaction with nature's wilds. It gives us a point of view by which we can see ourselves as being connected with the entire process of life," he says.

Although herbalism in the United States and Canada is only beginning to recover its lost prestige, other countries have successfully combined it with conventional medicine. In China, for example, traditional medicine that includes herbs is fully integrated into the nation's health care system, and natural remedies are used in nearly half of the cases treated there. In fact, only about 15 percent of the world's population has access to Western-style health care services. Most people in developing nations still rely on herbal treatments.

The World Health Organization, the United Nations agency that monitors health and health problems around the world, considers traditional medicine well-suited for the Third World for several reasons. It is less expensive than Western medicine, it is usually effective for local health problems, and it is already well-integrated into most Third World cultures. The first two of these reasons are arguments in favor of reintroducing herbalism into industrialized countries.

As public opinion begins to sway from complete faith in drugs, interest in herbs is increasing. Perhaps the day is not far off when the designations of traditional and modern medicine will have no significance, and all health care practitioners will feel comfortable working in a new system that incorporates both disciplines, Keville says.

What the Neanderthals Knew

The healing properties of plants have not changed. What was a healing herb a thousand years ago is still a healing herb. Today, we benefit from the accumulated herbal wisdom of the ages.

The plants that we know as healing herbs existed long before the first human appeared on Earth. No one knows how long it took for humans to discover the curative power of plants, but prehistoric sites in Iraq show that the Neanderthals used yarrow, marsh mallow, and other healing herbs some 60,000 years ago.

Prehistoric humans no doubt noticed that when animals appeared ill, they would often eat plants that they ordinarily ignored. Our ancestors sampled these plants and, in many cases, noticed curious effects, such as wakefulness, sleepiness, laxative action, and increased urination. The herbs that caused these effects were incorporated into prehistoric shamanism and later into medicine.

Observing animal behavior continues to point humanity to healing herbs today. Recently, naturalists at Tanzania's Gombe National Park noticed sick chimpanzees swallowing leaves from a bush called Aspilia. Subsequently, scientists discovered that Aspilia leaves contain a powerful antibiotic (thiarubrine-A).

The Sweet Smell of Successful Healing

Early humans were attracted to the aroma of healing herbs. They rubbed strong-smelling herbs on their bodies to repel insects and hide their human scent from animals that they feared or hunted. They also adorned themselves with sweet-smelling herbs to please their mates.

But foul odors, not fragrant ones, were key to the development of herbal healing. Early humans used plants such as rosemary, thyme, dill, and virtually all of today's culinary spices to mask the stench of rotting meats. Today, we use culinary herbs and spices only as flavor enhancers. But to our prehistoric ancestors, the flavor was incidental to food preservation.

Prehistoric humanity had no refrigeration, and meats spoiled quickly. Spoilage destroyed precious food reserves, and early humans learned through painful experience that eating rotten meats causes illness and sometimes death. No doubt, some prehistoric hunter or homemaker placed some rotting meat on a bed of wild mint, sage, basil, or other aromatic herb, hoping that its fragrance would mask the meat's nasty smell. It did, and amazingly, the meat didn't spoil as quickly.

A Little Knowledge and a Lot of Luck

Our ancestors also discovered many healing herbs simply by trial and error. They learned the hard way that some plants heal while others harm. They had little control over their world or their bodies. Their average life expectancy was barely 30 years. Because life was so full of threatening, often fatal, surprises, anything that made life more predictable acquired an aura of magic and healing.

Major herbal effects, such as vomiting or hallucinations, made big impressions, but prehistoric humans also recognized many herbs' more subtle healing benefits. We'll never know what possessed some ancient Chinese peasant to brew a tea from the small, ungainly stalks of the ma huang plant (Chinese ephedra). But 5,000 years ago, someone did and stumbled upon the world's oldest medicine, a decongestant. (Pseudo-ephedrine, a laboratory analog of ephedra, is still widely used in cold formulas.) Similarly, we'll never know how many roots the ancient scavengers dug up before they discovered ginger more than 4,000 years ago. Or why the Native Americans had a hunch that black cohosh might induce labor. But all over the world, ancient peoples dug, dried, chewed, pounded, rubbed, and brewed the plants around them, and through trial and error, they discovered the vast majority of healing herbs that we still use today.

Herbal trial and error becomes even more remarkable when we consider that cultures separated by thousands of miles arrived at similar uses for many healing herbs, apparently independently.

Herbal healing includes four major traditions: Chinese, Ayurvedic (in India), European (including Egyptian), and Native American. Until the fifteenth century, Old World cultures were isolated from the Americas. Nonetheless, Old and New World herbalists used many herbs similarly.

- Angelica and licorice: Asians, Europeans, and Native Americans all used these herbs to treat respiratory ailments.
- Hops and the mints: All the ancient herbal traditions used these herbs as stomach soothers.
- Blackberry and raspberry: These two popular herbs have been used around the world to treat diarrhea.
- White willow: All the herbal traditions used this herb to treat pain and inflammation.

During the nineteenth century, chemists used this "herbal convergence" to point them to the plants that provided extracts for the first pharmaceuticals. According to a report of the 121 prescription drugs derived from higher plants, about 74 percent came to the attention of drug companies because of their use in traditional herbal healing.

Shen Nung and the Classic of Herbs

The origins of Chinese herbalism are lost in the mists of time, but legend has it that around 3400 B.C., mythological emperor and sage Shen

Nung invented agriculture and discovered that many plants have medicinal value. He tested herbs on himself, recorded their effects, and died after consuming too much of one that was poisonous.

Chinese herbalists credit Shen Nung as author of China's first great herbal, the *Pen Tsao Ching ("Classic of Herbs")*, which listed 237 herbal prescriptions using dozens of herbs, including ephedra, rhubarb, and opium poppy. Succeeding emperors ordered new herbals, each more elaborate than the last. In 1590, Li Shih-Chen published his landmark 52-volume *Pen Tsao Kang Mu ("Catalog of Medicinal Herbs")*, listing 1,094 medicinal plants and an astounding 11,000 herbal formulas.

Starting in the mid-nineteenth century, European colonialists introduced Western medicine into China and dismissed traditional Chinese herbalism and acupuncture as nonsense. The Chinese felt the same way about the "foreign devils'" medicine, and the two systems seemed irreconcilable.

Shortly after the establishment of the People's Republic of China in 1949, the Chinese government decided that China's huge medically underserved population could benefit from the integration of Western and Chinese medicine. It hasn't been easy to combine these two systems, but nearly 50 years into the process, considerable progress has been made. In China today, Western-trained physicians practice alongside traditional herbalists and acupuncturists. Chinese and Western physicians examine the same patients, confer with each other, and often coordinate their recommendations.

A turning point in American acceptance of Chinese medicine occurred in 1972, when President Richard Nixon first visited China. Network news stations broadcast astonishing footage of a woman having abdominal surgery while fully conscious, her only anesthesia a few acupuncture needles in her earlobes and feet. Soon afterward, a columnist for the *New York Times* who had accompanied Nixon used acupuncture successfully to control his pain after an appendectomy. His first-person account in the nation's most influential newspaper helped open the United Sates to acupuncture and Chinese herbalism.

Jivaka and the Vedas

India's herbal tradition is almost as old as China's. It, too, has its legendary heroes. Around the time of the Hebrew Exodus from Egypt in approximately 1200 B.C., a poor young Indian named Jivaka wanted to study medicine. As the story goes, he approached the great Punarvasu Atreya, founder of India's first medical school. Jivaka had no money, so he offered to become Atreya's servant in exchange for medical training. After seven years he asked the great professor when his studies would be completed. Instead of answering, Atreya challenged him to search the countryside and collect all the plants that he considered medically useless. Jivaka did not return for many days. When he finally appeared, he was sullen and empty-handed. He told his mentor that he was unable to find a single plant without healing power. Professor Atreya replied, "Go! You now have the knowledge to be a physician." Ancient Indians called their medicine Ayurveda, from two Sanskrit words, *ayur*, "life," and *veda*, "knowledge." Ayurvedic medicine developed from the Vedas, India's four books of classic wisdom. The oldest, the 4,500-year-old *Rig-Veda*, contains astonishingly detailed descriptions of eye surgery, limb amputation, and formulas for medicines using 67 healing herbs, including ginger, cinnamon, and senna.

One herb that Ayurvedic healers introduced was rauwolfia. This plant is the source of reserpine, still used in Western medicine to manage high blood pressure.

After A.D. 600, Ayurvedic healing influenced Arab medicine, which combined Greco-Roman, Middle Eastern, and Asian therapies. Arab physicians in turn introduced some Ayurvedic practices into Europe.

During the nineteenth century, the British introduced Western medicine into India; however, an estimated 70 percent of Indians and Pakistanis still rely on Ayurvedic physicians and the healing herbs that they prescribe.

"The Stinking Ones" of the Nile

Although a hint of Chinese and Indian herbal tradition reached Europe by way of the Arabs, Western herbalism owes far more to another ancient land—Egypt. In 1874, in the Valley of the Tombs near Luxor, the German Egyptologist Georg Ebers discovered the world's oldest surviving medical text, a 65-foot papyrus dating from around 1500 B.C. The *Ebers Papyrus* summarized more than 1,000 years of ancient Egyptian medicine and listed 876 herbal formulas made from more than 500 plants, including about one-third of the herbs in today's Western pharmacopoeia.

Some of Ebers's formulas strike the modern reader as bizarre—for example, a shampoo made from a dog's paw, decayed palm leaves, and a donkey hoof, all boiled in oil, then rubbed on the head. But others sound surprisingly contemporary—for example, the recommendation to bandage moldy bread over wounds to prevent infection. Modern antibiotics are derived from molds.

But the Egyptians' affection for fragrant herbs paled next to their obsession with two herbs that many ancients considered foul-smelling: garlic and onions. The Egyptians believed that garlic and onions strengthened the body and prevented disease (a view supported by modern science). They ate so much that the Greek historian Herodotus called them the stinking ones. (In fact, six cloves of garlic were found in the tomb of King Tut.)

By about 500 B.C., Egyptian herbalists were considered the finest in the Mediterranean, and the rulers from Rome to Babylon recruited them as court physicians. Aspiring physicians, including many from Rome and among them Galen, went to Egypt to study with the medical masters of the Nile. Thus, Egyptian herbal healing began to influence Western medicine.

European Herbal Healers (and Assassins)

Roman herbalists were as likely to be killers as healers. The imperial court of the Roman Empire bubbled with intrigue as hostile factions plotted murder to gain political power. Among assassination methods—knifing, "accidents," and poisoning—the herbal approach was most popular. Death occurred some time after the deed, allowing for escape or alibi. And in an age before autopsy, when apparently healthy people often sickened and died suddenly, wily poisoners might escape unsuspected. As a result, rulers throughout the Roman Empire were obsessed with the identification of herbal poisons and the development of antidotes.

When Rome fell, the barbarians seized not only Rome's lands and wealth but also its vast stores of herbs and spices. During one attack, the barbarians demanded horses and money—and 3,000 pounds of black pepper.

After the fall of Rome, European medicine was dominated by the Catholic Church, which officially viewed illness as punishment from God and treatable only by prayer and penance. Unofficially, however, Catholic monks preserved Greco-Roman herbalism by copying the ancient texts.

Among the monastic orders, the Benedictines were the most avid herbalists. They were the first Europeans to adopt the Arab practice of transferring the healing power of herbs to alcohol. They flavored wine with digestion-promoting herbs and created the forerunners of today's liqueurs, one of which still bears the order's name.

Charlemagne, emperor of the Holy Roman Empire, was so impressed by the Benedictines' herb gardens, he ordered all the monasteries in his vast realm to plant "physic gardens" to ensure an adequate supply of healing herbs. Charlemagne called herbs friends of the physician and cook.

The most notable Benedictine herbalist was Hildegard of Bingen, a twelfth-century abbess of the Rupertsburg Convent in the German Rhineland. A nun from age 15, Hildegard claimed that visions of God commanded her to treat the sick and compile her herbal formulas. Her book, *Hildegard's Medicine*, combined mystical Catholicism and early German folk medicine with her own extensive experience using herbs.

Hildegard was unique. She wrote an original medical work at a time when the few Europeans who were literate—mostly monks—contented themselves with copying the Greeks and Romans. Some of Hildegard's advice sounds silly. For poor vision she advocated rubbing the eyes with a topaz soaked in wine. But many of her recommendations were quite sensible. She advocated a balanced diet and tooth brushing with aloe and myrrh, both of which have antibacterial, decay-preventing properties.

Around the time when the Benedictines invented liqueur, Germanic Angles and Saxons were settling in England. They brought European herbalism with them and learned how the native Celts and their priests, the Druids, used healing herbs. Around A.D. 950, a nobleman named Bald persuaded England's King Alfred to commission the first British herbal. The book combined Anglo-Saxon and Celtic herbalism with Greco-Roman and Arab practices. Called the *Leech Book of Bald*, it discussed 500 plants, including vervain and mistletoe, both sacred to the Druids.

Wise Women: From Healers to Witches

Hildegard of Bingen was lucky that she lived when she did. If she had practiced herbalism from 1300 to 1650, then she probably would have been burned at the stake as a witch.

It's not clear what caused Europe's 350 years of witch-hunts. Feminists link them to the rise of secular medicine as a male-dominated profession. Others blame the witch-hunts on the bubonic plague, or the Black Death, which swept Europe in waves and killed half of its population.

Whatever the cause, after 1300, the image of the female folk herbalist changed from wise woman to witch. The witch-hunts started in Germany and eventually reached all of Europe. Accusations of "sexual intercourse with the devil" were typically accompanied by testimony that the alleged witch practiced herbal medicine and made healing mixtures, cosmetics, love potions, aphrodisiacs, abortion-inducing preparations, and poisons.

Accusations of poisoning were particularly damning. It's quite possible that some women herbalists continued the Roman tradition of herbal assassination. But this was the era before the discovery of the "dose-response relationship"—the idea that the greater the dose, the greater the effect. Many so-called witches' plants, poisonous in large amounts, cause no harm in therapeutic or cosmetic amounts.

The witch-hunts failed to eradicate women's herbalism, but they succeeded in driving it underground. More than a century after the last witch-hunts, the old woman who helped popularize foxglove—the source of the heart drug digitalis—said it was a secret family recipe. Her forebears had good reason to keep it secret.

Sickly Colonists, Robust Natives

Europeans considered America's natives ignorant savages—except when it came to health and healing. Explorers and colonists were all too familiar with the plagues, pestilence, and suffering back home. They marveled at the Native Americans' good health, physical stamina, and fine teeth. Not surprisingly, colonists became eager students of their herbal medicine.

Puritan Boston minister/physician Cotton Mather wrote that Native American healers produced "many cures that are truly stupendous." And when John Wesley, founder of Methodism, visited America in the 1730s, he wrote that the Native Americans had "exceedingly few" diseases, and that their medicines were "quick and generally infallible." Later, even those in the military who hated the natives marveled at the effectiveness of their wound treatments. And many early American physicians touted their apprenticeship to Native American herbalists.

Of course, America's native healers also had their critics, mostly among university-trained physicians. Philadelphia doctor Benjamin Rush, a signer of the Declaration of Independence, declared, "We have no discoveries in the materia medica . . . from the Indians. It would be a reproach to our schools of physic if modern physicians were not more successful than Indians."

How wrong Rush was. Native Americans introduced White settlers to many valuable healing herbs, including black and blue cohosh, black haw, boneset, cascara sagrada, echinacea, chaparral, goldenseal, lobelia, Oregon grape, sarsaparilla, slippery elm, wild cherry, and witch hazel.

Of course, American colonists grew both culinary and medicinal herbs in their kitchen gardens. Thomas Jefferson was a typical herb grower. His 1,000-square-foot garden at Monticello contained 26 herbs.

Thomson's Botanic Medicine

Early America's leading herbalist was Samuel Thomson. Born in Alstead, New Hampshire, in 1760, he studied with a midwife and Native American healers. Around 1800, his daughter became seriously ill. Unsure of his skills, Thomson called a physician, who pronounced her incurable. Then Thomson cured her with herbs and hot baths inspired by Native American sweat lodges. Soon after, he declared himself a doctor.

Thomson detested the "regular" physicians of his day, who relied on bleeding, violent laxatives, and mercury. These treatments were called heroic medicine, but the only heroes were the patients. Consider the case of George Washington. One day in 1799, the elderly but otherwise healthy Father of Our Country developed a sore throat with a fever and chills. Chances are that he had strep throat or some other minor infection, which probably would have cleared up with rest, hot liquids, and herbal antibiotics such as garlic and onion. Instead, Washington's heroic physicians bled him of 4 pints of blood, leaving him anemic and weak, then gave him laxatives and mercury. He was dead within 24 hours.

In 1839, at the height of his popularity, Thomson claimed three million adherents. This was probably an exaggeration, but there's no doubt that Thomsonian herbalism was enormously popular. Thomson boasted that half of Ohio practiced his herbal healing, but his critics said that only a third did.

After Thomson's death in 1843, his medical system fell from fashion. Some practitioners, the naturopaths, continued the Thomsonian herb/bath tradition. One was Dr. John Kellogg of Battle Creek, Michigan, an American physician who invented the nation's first health food, the cornflake, and founded Kellogg's cereal company. But Thomsonian medicine was largely replaced by homeopathy and eclectic herbalism.

The Eclectics: America's Scientific Herbalists

Despite the "regular" physicians' reliance on bleeding, violent laxatives, and mercury, most nineteenth-century medicines were herbal. In 1820, two-thirds of the treatments in the *U.S. Pharmacopoeia* were botanical. In 1880, the figure was almost three-quarters.

In the 1820s, a group of antiheroic practitioners—Thomsonians, herbalists trained by the Native Americans, and disillusioned "regulars"—created the Reformed Medical Society to promote antiheroic, largely herbal healing. In 1830, the Society met in New York City to found a Reformed medical school.

They adopted the term *eclectic* to describe their herb-based approach, which combined European, Asian, Native American, and slave herbalism.

The Eclectics were scientific herbalists. They experimented with herbs, analyzed them chemically, extracted their active constituents, published their findings in scientific journals, and were prominent in the early pharmaceutical industry.

The years from 1880 to 1900 marked the heyday of Eclectic medicine. Its practitioners numbered about 8,000. But Eclectic popularity declined in the twentieth century to the point that the period from 1920 though the 1960s might be called the lost decades of herbal healing. Medical schools ignored herbs. Pharmaceutical drugs replaced herbal tinctures in the nation's pharmacies. Even many culinary herbs fell from popularity. But herbal healing didn't die. It simply reverted to what it had been for most of its history: folk medicine practiced by women and men who grew and gathered their own herbs and prescribed them as the classic herbals recommended.

Let the Herbal Renaissance Begin

Starting in the late 1960s, many Americans began changing their attitudes about health and healing. They decided to invest their energy in preventing illness, rather than treating it after the fact. One step in that direction was a retreat from salt as the nation's main seasoning because of research linking it to high blood pressure, heart disease, and stroke. Many Americans retired their saltshakers and rediscovered culinary herbs and spices.

Today herbal products line the shelves in health food stores and supermarkets. Authorities estimate that retail sales of healing herbs, kitchen spices, herb books, herbal teas, and herbal cosmetics and personal-care products top $3 billion a year.

The herbal healing boom involves the convergence of many trends including the following:

Increased interest in self-care. Mainstream medicine has produced miracles, but it has also grown expensive and impersonal. To save time, money, and limit their dependence on doctors, many Americans have turned to prevention and self-care. Healing herbs fit neatly into lifestyles focused on sound nutrition, fitness, and stress management.

Increased interest in alternative healing arts. Homeopathy, naturopathy, and Chinese and Ayurvedic medicines have become more popular in recent years. These healing arts use herbal medicines.

Reaction against high technology. The very wizardry of high technology creates a yearning for more down-to-earth approaches to human problems. When there is a choice, many Americans prefer healing herbs to the pharmaceuticals often derived from them.

Increased environmental consciousness. Pollution, industrial development, and the destruction of tropical rain forests are causing record numbers of plant extinctions. As a result, scientists are scrambling to preserve our plant heritage and screen new herbs as potential medicines. Several years ago, the Drug Research and Development Branch of the National Cancer Institute (NCI) launched an ambitious project to test plants for anti-cancer activity. NCI scientists have investigated 70,000 extracts from 7,500 species and have found 750 with anti-tumor effects. But much work remains. Of the estimated 250,000 plant species on Earth, scientists estimate that only about 15 percent have been screened for medicinal uses.

But even as these screenings move forward, it's clear that the world's oldest medicines, the herbs that humanity has used for thousands of years, will continue to play a key role in health and healing as the twentieth century becomes the twenty-first.

The Healthy Harvest

Most herbs are easy to grow, either in backyard gardens or simply in flowerpots on the windowsill. But to preserve their healing powers, you have to dry and store them properly. Here's how.

Sure, it's quicker, easier, and sometimes safer to simply buy herbal medicines. But in doing so, you forgo the exercise and miss the spiritual power of planting, nurturing, harvesting, processing, and preparing your own green medicines.

Foraging for wild herbs, for instance, creates a spiritual connection to the plant and the forest where it grows. Known as wildcrafting in botanical lingo, foraging has a therapeutic power that more than compensates for the loss of exactness you would find in store-bought herbs, says James A. Duke, Ph.D., a retired U.S. Department of Agriculture botanist and author of *The Green Pharmacy*.

Of course, picking wild medicinal herbs can be hazardous, and you don't want to try it unless you can positively identify the plants that you're selecting. Dr. Duke, for instance, recalls one elderly couple traveling out West who mistook foxglove for comfrey. Unfortunately, foxglove is the source of the heart-stimulating drug digitalis, and it had fatal consequences.

So, if you aren't really familiar with field botany, harvesting wild plants probably isn't a wise choice, Dr. Duke advises. But if you know what you're doing, in just about any part of the United States, you can harvest a bounty of useful medicinal herbs just by stepping out your front door.

If you're not familiar with herbs at first, you can have a good deal of fun finding out more about them. Most metropolitan areas have botanical organizations—museum groups, scout groups, hiking clubs, or university extension departments—that offer classes in the identification of local edible and medicinal plants. And hiking, Dr. Duke says, is much more fun when you can munch your way along the trail.

Growing Windowsill Wonders

Like wildcrafting, growing your own herbs gives you the raw material that you need to create potent natural remedies. But it also gives you an even deeper spiritual connection to your medicines than foraging, according to Dr. Duke. No matter what you grow, gardening is a therapeutic, self-empowering hobby. And from what we know about mind-body medicine, self-grown herbal medicines should work better than anything store-bought or foraged, he says.

All you need is a kitchen windowsill where you can grow a potted aloe plant—your instant herbal emergency kit in case of accidental burns. (Just snip off a leaf, slit it open, and apply the yellow-green inner-leaf gel to the burn.) There are many other herbs that you can raise on a windowsill or on your back porch. If you're a city dweller, you can find space in a roof garden, courtyard, or balcony. Quite a few medicinal/culinary species that are native to semi-arid climates will also flourish on sunny kitchen windowsills. Here are some to consider.

Basil. This insect-repelling herb is recommended for treating bad breath and headaches.

Chives. Along with their cousins, garlic and onions, chives help prevent cancer and treat high blood pressure.

Dill. This is deservedly famous as a remedy for colic and gas.

Fennel. This herb is good for treating upset stomach as well as indigestion.

Hyssop. Mentioned in the Bible, hyssop contains several antiviral compounds and is useful in treating herpes. (It's under review as an AIDS therapy.)

Lavender. Some varieties of this lovely herb are loaded with sedative compounds that can penetrate the skin. Toss a handful into your bathwater if you want a nice-smelling way to relax.

Parsley. Best known as a great source of chlorophyll for combating bad breath, parsley is rich in the mineral zinc—good for men's reproductive health.

Peppermint. This is a major source of cooling, soothing, stomach-settling menthol.

Rosemary. This tasty culinary spice is rich in antioxidants and is a useful treatment for Alzheimer's disease.

Sage. Sage shares much of the medicinal potential of rosemary.

Savory. Europeans add this herb to bean dishes to reduce flatulence.

Thyme. One of the best sources of thymol—an antiseptic, stomach-soothing compound that helps prevent the internal blood clots that cause heart attack.

Cultivate Your Own Pharmacy

On 6 acres in Fulton, Maryland, Dr. Duke grows some 200 species of herbs, most of them medicinal. During the growing season one of his great pleasures in life is to stroll the grounds and check on all the plants.

Almost hourly, when spending the day at the computer, he takes breaks and visits his herb garden. During his strolls he often harvests aromatic mints for hot mint tea on a cool morning or iced mint tea on a hot afternoon.

Learning to grow herbs outdoors is easy, Dr. Duke says. Here are a few of his favorites.

Chastetree. A perennial flowering shrub, it has a berry that may be very beneficial in normalizing hormones during a woman's menopausal changes.

Goldenseal. This antibiotic herb is best grown in shade.

Lemon balm. Also known as Melissa, this weedy antiviral mint has sedative properties. Though it sometimes looks like it has died away, it always comes back.

Mountain mint. This is an insect-repelling herb that should be more popular among gardeners than it is.

Oregano. This is another weedy mint, and it's a great source of antioxidants.

Self-heal. The reputation of this mint as a panacea is only slightly exaggerated.

Spearmint. This herb is about as good as peppermint for settling the stomach.

St.-John's-wort. This is the best herbal treatment for depression.

Valerian. The roots contain a great anxiety-relieving sedative. But be warned—the tea smells like dirty gym socks.

Wild yam. Many herbalists recommend this herb for women's reproductive health.

Willow. This is a tree with an easy-peeling bark that contains the herbal version of aspirin.

Harvesting Your Herbal Bounty

Okay, so you have a big peppermint patch—or whatever—growing in your garden or on your windowsill. Now what?

First you must harvest your herbs. You can snip off leaves and use them as needed. In fact, the more you clip the leaves of medicinal plants, the more medicinal they become. This makes sense botanically because the medicinal constituents of herbs are basically part of the plant's self-protection system. Harvesting the leaves makes the plant respond as if it's under attack (which it is), so it produces more of what protects it. Studies have shown that infections, insect infestations, and leaf plucking, among other attacks on the plant, increase the levels of some chemicals that we view as medicines.

Though herbalists argue for harvesting herbs early in the morning while there is still dew on them, Dr. Duke disagrees. Early-morning harvests dilute your herb with water, meaning that your herb has proportionately more water and less chemical until it's dried. Instead, he contends that you get the greatest concentration of plant chemicals and the least amount of water when you collect leaves during a hot, dry day, but before the leaves have wilted.

Roots are best collected in spring or fall. Bark may be collected in spring, especially if the compounds that you seek are in the living bark. If you're collecting seeds for food, Dr. Duke recommends that you get them before they have dried out and hardened. But if you're harvesting them to plant next year rather than using them for medicine immediately, you should wait until they've dried out.

Feel free to use herbs fresh, especially in cooking. Fresh culinary herbs and spices always taste best. (When harvesting fresh culinary herbs that are to be used right away, Dr. Duke generally uses a plastic bag to help retain the moisture.

Preserving the Goods

If you intend to preserve your herbs for future use, then it's best to dry them. Collect clean, unblemished leaves and stems in a brown paper bag rather than a plastic bag and write the plant's name and the collection date on the outside of the bag.

If you don't stuff the bag too tightly, many herbs can be dried right in the paper bag. Try to make a run through your herb garden with paper bags before the last killing frost, collecting herbs for winter medicines, soups, and teas, Dr. Duke recommends.

Check your brown-bagged herbs after about a week, and if they are not drying—becoming papery and crumbly—spread them out in a dry, shaded area on newspapers or on a clean piece of wood or screen so that they can dry before mildew attacks. Discard all of the herbs in the batch if any of them develop a white, powdery film or black spots on the surface or if they become soggy or rotten.

Once dried, herbs can be kept in paper bags or stuffed into plastic bags, says Dr. Duke. You can also use glass jars with lids.

When it comes to success in drying, a great deal depends on your local weather conditions. In arid weather, herbs may dry too rapidly, especially in direct sunlight. In humid and especially in foggy weather, you may have to use heat, baking your herbs in an oven to get the moisture out. Here are some helpful hints to get you started.

- When drying leaves or flowers, tie small bunches of the herbs together and hang them upside down in a dry, well-ventilated area, such as an attic or large pantry. To prevent them from getting dusty, you can hang the herbs inside paper bags with holes punched in the sides to allow air to circulate. Be careful not to crush the herbs, since this will cause the precious oils to dissipate.
- When drying roots, cut them into thin pieces, thread them on a length of string, and hang them to dry.
- When drying seeds, hang the entire plant upside down in a paper bag and allow it to dry. As the plant dries, the seeds will fall to the bottom of the bag.
- Light, heat, and oxygen are the enemies of herb potency, so store your herbs in a cool, dark place, like a cellar or cupboard far from any heat source. To minimize the oxygen around stored herbs, fill your containers as full as possible and move the herbs to smaller

containers as you use them up. Properly stored dried herbs can last for several months or even several years depending on the herb. Herbs that are still useful should smell and taste like the original herb and have strong color.

The Green Grocery

The ads promise wonders. Your common sense urges caution. How to start? Here are some important buying guidelines for every herbal enthusiast.

Herbal medicine is hot in the United States today for a variety of reasons, including the often-erroneous belief that things organic or natural are inherently better, says Varro E. Tyler, Ph.D., Sc.D., former professor of pharmacognosy at Purdue University in West Lafayette, Indiana, and author of *The New Honest Herbal* and *Herbs of Choice*.

Herbs are generally milder in their actions and produce fewer significant side effects than synthetic drugs. They may also cost less. Some of them produce therapeutic results not obtainable with synthetic drugs. The immune-stimulating effect of echinacea in shortening the duration of the common cold is a prime example. And many herbs have several active ingredients that work together to produce an effect that could not be realized with a single synthetic drug.

Under current U.S. laws and regulations most herbs, or botanicals, are sold as dietary supplements (foods), not as approved drugs, so label claims of therapeutic value are forbidden. It's possible to include a statement about the effect of the product on the structure or function of the human body ("for the brain" or "for the nervous system," for instance), but these remarks are often so vague that they are meaningless, Dr. Tyler says. If such a statement is made, it must be followed by another statement indicating that the claim has not been evaluated by the Food and Drug Administration. Then, yet another sentence must appear noting that the product is not intended to diagnose, treat, cure, or prevent any disease. Of course, that's exactly why you would buy the herb in the first place, so it all becomes a bit ridiculous—and more than a little hypocritical, Dr. Tyler points out.

Product literature included with the product package can legally give additional information if it is scientifically accurate, balanced, truthful, and generic—that is, not referring to a brand-name product. The trouble is, there's no system in place to monitor compliance with these regulations, and few retailers are falling over themselves to present the negative features—like side effects—of the products that they sell, Dr. Tyler says.

So take a hard look at products that sound too good to be true. Do not trust product literature as fact, warns Kathi Keville, director of the American Herb Association and author of *Herbs for Health and Healing*. As with other commodities, herbal advertising sometimes stretches the truth, uses tricky wording, or tells only part of the story. Most herb companies claim that their products and processing techniques are the very best. They probably believe this, but that doesn't mean it's true.

Once You Buy Herbs, Treat 'Em Right

As with any plant, a number of factors can influence the potency of herbs, including growing conditions, harvesting method, drying and storage processes, even the time of year and time of day when the herbs were harvested. Don't underestimate freshness—the moment an herb is picked, enzymes released in the plant begin to break down its active compounds. Light, heat, and air all increase oxidation, which causes herbs to deteriorate.

Store herbs in airtight containers, preferably glass, away from heat and direct sunlight. Herbs in large pieces will keep longer than those that are finely cut or powdered. Plan on keeping leaves and flowers for at least two years, roots and barks for three years. Since there is no exact cutoff date, use an herb's color, taste, and aroma as guides to tell you how much potency remains. Even after it is dried, an herb should retain its taste and color, and a fragrant plant should still have its characteristic aroma. If your herbs ever develop a white powdery film, black spots, or a foul smell, discard them.

Making Sense of the Hype

One of the major problems in using herbs intelligently is the fact that the U.S. government has no quality standards for them. So it's difficult for consumers to be sure that they're actually getting quality products that conform to labeled specifications, Dr. Tyler says. Here are a few hints that should help.

Grab the new kid off the shelf. Many botanicals, especially those containing volatile oils, have a short shelf life—about three to six months—and deteriorate with age, Dr. Tyler says. Some, such as feverfew, should definitely be stored in a refrigerator, both in the store and at home, but you won't find that information on the label. Although an herb's shelf life can vary, expiration dates on some packages can give you a clue about the freshness of the product.

Use all of your senses. One potential problem is that the herbs used by some manufacturers may be of poor quality. Manufacturers get away with this because it can be difficult for the consumer to determine the quality of pills. If you're trying out a new brand, or want to quickly check the quality of one you're using, there's a simple procedure that can help. Open a capsule or mash a tablet with the back of a spoon, then smell and examine the powder. The herbs inside should still carry the color, fragrance, and taste of the original plant, Keville says. For example, if dried chamomile looks brown instead of yellow, or if you cannot detect much of the characteristic fragrance in peppermint, these herbs are probably not good. Try another brand or variety the next time you buy.

Tinctures are born travelers. If you have wanderlust, buy tinctures, suggests Michael Castleman, author of *Nature's Cures*. Tinctures stay potent longer than bulk herbs or tea bags, and their concentrations make them compact—good for travel or conserving shelf space in medicine cabinets.

Teas and Tinctures

Herbs are only worthwhile if they are properly prepared.
Here's a quick primer on how to get the best results.

An herbalist's definition of an herb differs from that of a botanist. The botanist defines an herbaceous plant as one with a fleshy stem that dies back in the winter. The herbalist, however, considers all medicinal and cosmetic plants as herbs. This broad definition of herbs includes trees, shrubs, mushrooms, lichens, and, of course, fruits and vegetables that have medicinal properties. In many of the recipes in this chapter, you will find items that you consider food rather than herbs, such as apple juice or shiitake mushrooms.

There are countless different herbs and combinations of herbs that are used for health and healing. But even the most potent herb can become worthless if not properly prepared. Fortunately, there are only a few basic kinds of preparations that are used in treating illnesses and wounds herbally; these are the delivery systems for the healing powers of herbs.

These preparations transform dried or fresh herbs into something that can be taken internally, such as a tea or capsule, or applied externally, as in a skin salve or a massage oil. In many cases more than one preparation is applicable for a specific treatment, says Kathi Keville, director of the American Herb Association and author of *Herbs for Health and Healing*.

Some preparations, such as tinctures and body oils, can be made from either fresh or dried herbs. The best method for extracting an herb's properties varies from herb to herb. For example, Saint-John's-wort, oat berries, and feverfew lose most of their properties when dried. A significant portion of the essential oils in fragrant herbs such as peppermint and chamomile is lost in even the most careful drying process. On the other hand, herbs that contain a great deal of water—comfrey and calendula flowers, for example—are sometimes best when used in dried form; otherwise, the final product will be too diluted, Keville says.

Most of these preparations can be bought ready-made from health food stores—either as individual herbs or in blends of several different herbs. If you feel ambitious enough to make your own concoction, Keville has developed a number of recipes. When deciding which preparation is the most suitable for you, consider availability, cost, convenience, and of course, effectiveness.

Many herbal recipes use as their basic ingredient not herbs but essential oils derived from herbs. These oils carry many medicinal properties of the herbs from which they are extracted. They are easy to use but are also highly concentrated, so they must be diluted and used moderately to prevent overdoses. As a result, they are mostly used externally. Do not confuse essential oils with vegetable oils such as olive oil, which are used as carrier oils in skin products.

Treatments are divided into internal preparations and external preparations, as the nature of the ailment generally determines the nature of the treatment.

Preparations for Internal Use

The following preparations are designed to be taken internally. Included in the descriptions are definitions—for example, what makes a tincture a tincture—basic directions, and average doses.

Tinctures

Tinctures, also called herbal extracts, are a concentrated liquid form of herbal medicine. A tincture is easy to carry, easily assimilated, and needs no refrigeration. It will keep for years, another important consideration for anyone with an on-the-go lifestyle. This concentrated form of herbs makes it easier to down strong-tasting herbs or take large doses. In fact, because a tincture is so concentrated, it is best to dilute it into an instant tea by adding it to water or juice; the average dose is about 30 drops, ¼ teaspoon, or half a dropperful (based on the 1-ounce droppers used for most commercially available tinctures). Certain tinctures are used externally, mostly as skin antiseptics. All tinctures take effect quite quickly.

The liquid medium of a tincture is alcohol. The alcohol draws important properties from the herb (or herbs), leaving behind the more inactive substances, such as starch or cellulose. It also extracts compounds that are not water-soluble. This means that a few herbs, such as goldenseal and black cohosh, and gums such as myrrh, are stronger when made into tinctures. Making a tincture requires no heat, so essential oils are retained.

One ounce of tincture contains about 600 drops or 6 teaspoons, which equals about 20 doses per bottle. Price-wise, that's about 35 to 40 cents a dose. This means that tinctures are more costly than teas, but most people don't mind paying for the convenience. When using the herbs suggested in this book, it is not necessary to use the exact number of drops; estimating is fine. (Remember, we are talking about very safe herbs, not drugstore pharmaceuticals.)

A tincture is much easier to get down than a strong-tasting tea. Keville finds tinctures to be handy for dispensing herbs to children and animals as well as reluctant adults.

If you have religious, health, or other objections to using alcohol, tinctures may not be for you. Otherwise, do not be concerned; many doctors consider a small amount of alcohol healthy and an aid to digestion, Keville says. A typical four doses a day totals less than ½ teaspoon of alcohol. Studies show that most people can handle 6 to 12 times that amount, unless they have liver problems. If you prefer, you can eliminate much of the alcohol by dropping a dose of tincture into a cup of boiling water. That alcohol evaporates, leaving the medicine behind. Do this with only one dose at a time, since the tincture will spoil without alcohol to preserve it, Keville says.

Do not confuse herbal tinctures with homeopathic remedies or flower essences, which are used differently. Although all three products are preserved with alcohol and sold in the same type of dropper bottle, homeopathic remedies and flower essences are so dilute that there is often no detectable trace of the original herbs in them. Remember that these products are not interchangeable; each has different effects, Keville says.

There are a number of variations on the tincture theme, and this often makes it very confusing for the consumer. To make matters worse, these terms are used loosely and sometimes interchangeably. These definitions should help.

Concentrated liquid extract. This is a tincture that has had most of its water and alcohol removed, making it a thick, semisolid that can be blended into pills or reconstituted with glycerin or alcohol into a liquid preparation. This is one way to make alcohol-free tinctures.

Double extraction. This is a double-strength tincture that is made by making a regular tincture, straining out the herbs, then combining that tincture with a fresh batch of herbs to make a second tincture. Because twice as much time and twice as much work are required to make a double extraction, only a few herb companies bother with this method.

Standardized or guaranteed extract. This product, usually a tincture or pill, is guaranteed to contain a specified quantity of the herb's main active compound. Laboratory tests are used to determine the amount of an active ingredient in an herb. If that quantity is lower than what is guaranteed on the label, that herb is rejected and one that meets this requirement is used in its place. In a few cases, such as with the herb ephedra, a purified amount of the active ingredient is added to increase potency to the stated level. To achieve this, certain important compounds are isolated and others are often discarded. Some herbalists refuse to use herbs that have been altered in this way, but many laboratory scientists prefer them for their consistent strength.

USP standardized. Until tinctures began to be replaced by synthetic drugs following World War I, they were commonly sold in pharmacies and were made according to proportions set down in the U.S. Pharmacopoeia (USP), the pharmacist's guidebook. Today, few herbal companies can afford pharmaceutical licenses, and herbs in general cannot legally be advertised or sold as specific medicines. Because manufacturing methods and herb qualities vary, products often have different strengths, even when they come from the same company. These traditional USP standards are still used by some companies.

Glycerites

Glycerites are syrupy liquids that provide an alcohol-free alternative to the more popular tincture in which an herb's properties are extracted using alcohol. A glycerite is created using glycerin in place of alcohol. Glycerin has a sweet taste, but it does not affect blood sugar like honey, sugar, and other sweets do. In fact, a well-known nineteenth-century American herbalist and doctor of naturopathic medicine, Edward E. Shook, preferred glycerites for most of his medicines.

There are two types of glycerin. One type, derived from animal fat, is a by-product of soap making; the other is derived from vegetable oil. Although soap itself is not edible, glycerin is. It is even used in some foods, such as frosting and baked goods, to hold ingredients together and keep them moist. Animal-fat glycerin is sold in pharmacies. Vegetable glycerin can be ordered through health food stores. A synthetic glycerin derived from petroleum is becoming increasingly popular.

An average glycerite dose is about 30 drops, ¼ teaspoon, or half a dropperful (based on the 1-ounce droppers used for most commercially available tinctures). This dosage should be diluted in water, tea, or juice, as it may irritate your mouth otherwise, Keville says. Glycerites are not as potent as tinctures and are more expensive than tea. Like tinctures, however, they are easy to carry and to make preparations from. For instance, a glycerite can be used to make instant tea. They also make a great base for syrups, and they have a long shelf life.

Pills

Tablets and capsules release their herbal contents in the stomach as they dissolve. They provide an easy way to down herbs, as long as you don't mind swallowing pills. They are slower-acting and generally less potent than tinctures, but like glycerites, they do not contain alcohol. They certainly offer a faster and more convenient method of treatment than tea—which has to be prepared—and they allow you to avoid tasting unpalatable herbs. They are more expensive than tea because you pay for the convenience of having the herb powdered, processed, bottled, and marketed. For most users the convenience outweighs the expense. Compact and easiest to carry of any herbal preparation, they are very handy in a traveling herbal first-aid kit. When carefully stored in a cool place, they last for at least a year.

Since capsules are a popular way to take herbs, you will find a large selection available at health food stores and some pharmacies. (Powdered liquid extracts, tinctures, or freeze-dried herbs are sometimes put into capsules or tablets. Because they are so concentrated, they are usually mixed with a filler to give them more bulk.)

Capsules and tablets do have some disadvantages beyond cost, Keville says. Many herbalists feel that the body better assimilates an herb that has been tasted. Bitters, for example, stimulate digestive juices when tasted. Indeed, what a surprise it must be when your stomach gets hit with a bitter herb such as goldenseal without any advance warning from the taste buds.

If you want to fill your own capsules—either to save money or because you can't find the herbal formula you want—you can buy empty capsules at health food stores. This, however, is a tedious job, Keville says. It involves powdering the herbs, scooping them into the capsule, and packing them in with a chopstick or similar tool. You can speed the process along by using one of several types of capping machines sold through health food stores.

The typical tablet or capsule is roughly comparable to ½ cup of tea or ⅙ ounce of herb, Keville says. Consult the product label for dosage.

Syrups

A syrup is a tincture, liquid extract, glycerite, or sometimes a strong tea that is sweetened and thickened with sugar, honey, glycerin, molasses, rice syrup, or fruit syrup. (*Caution*: Doctors warn that you should not give honey to children under two years of age.) Glycerin is often preferred since it will not ferment like honey. A syrup makes an ideal cough remedy because it coats and soothes the throat, Keville says.

While syrups are tasty, easy to carry, and long-lasting, the added sweeteners in them can pose a problem for people who have blood sugar problems, such as diabetes and hypoglycemia. If you have one of these disorders, avoid syrups, Keville warns. The other potential problem with syrups is that their herbal content is often low because of overdilution. The average dose of a syrup is 1 tablespoon.

Teas

Teas offer one of the simplest and least expensive ways to prepare herbs. In fact, a cup of tea usually costs only a few cents, and the typical dose is 1 teaspoon of herb per cup, 1 cup three or four times daily. Making tea can help you become familiar with the herbs as you feel, smell, and taste them. Relaxing for a few minutes while you drink your medicine is a healthy way to remind yourself to slow down, Keville says. Some remedies—for example, many fever-reducing teas and some diurectics—work only when taken as hot tea because the heat promotes sweating.

Teas have their advantages, but you may find that you don't have time to make them every day. Of course, drinking tea sounds like a great idea—until you brew up some foul-tasting herbs, then try to drink them a few times a day. Teas can also be a problem if you have to lug a Thermos around with you. Refrigerated teas will keep for a couple of days.

There are several different methods of preparing teas.

Infusions. These are made by pouring hot water over herbs and steeping for 5 to 10 minutes in a saucepan, teapot, or cup. Flowers and leaves are the usual ingredients. Commercial herb teas that come in tea bags are cut extra fine to produce tea quickly, usually in 5 minutes. To retain heat-sensitive essential oils contained in the herbs, cover the pot or pan.

Decoctions. These are prepared by gently simmering herbs in water for 15 to 30 minutes. The most common ingredients in decoctions are roots and bark. The Chinese prefer to simmer root and bark teas even longer. The high heat releases more properties from heavy barks and roots than steeping does. Keep the heat very low when simmering aromatic roots such as valerian, elecampane, and angelica so that their essential oils aren't lost into the air. Some barks and roots can be brewed a second time.

Cold Infusions. These are made by soaking herbs in cold water for about 8 hours. Because this method takes such a long time, it is generally reserved for delicate, fragrant herbs that lose their essential oils when heated.

Two modern versions of tea are increasingly finding their way to market. Flavor-enhanced tea has essential oils or flavorings—such as almond, mint, cinnamon, or citrus—added to increase its flavor. Instant tea is made using herbs that have been quickly dried in a high-heat chamber. This removes their water but retains most of their properties and flavor, making the tea very concentrated. Instant tea is then added to a substance that dissolves easily, such as lactose or dextrin, to increase its bulk.

Vinegars

Herbal vinegars are prepared like tinctures, but the herbs are infused into vinegar instead of into alcohol. Though vinegar does not draw out an herb's properties as well as alcohol, herbal vinegars offer the convenience of a tincture without the alcohol. Because most herbal vinegars are designed for culinary use, they are not medicinal strength. Also, the selection is limited. An herbal vinegar is easy to take, provided that you like the taste of vinegar, and it can be used surreptitiously in a meal as salad dressing or in any recipe calling for vinegar. The typical dose is 1 to 2 teaspoons. Herbal vinegar also makes a fine sore-throat gargle. In addition, it can be used externally as a hair rinse or as a skin wash for fungal infections.

Caution: Vinegar eats away at tooth enamel, so be sure to rinse your mouth thoroughly after drinking it.

Preparations for External Use

The following preparations are designed to be used externally. Included in the descriptions are definitions—for instance, what is a compress—as well as basic directions.

Aromatic Waters

Scented waters are used to treat many different skin problems ranging from acne to burns. They can also be used for purely cosmetic purposes. Because the essential oils they contain are so dilute, aromatic waters can be applied directly to the skin and taken internally. They also come in handy for soaking herbal compresses to treat skin and complexion problems. But they are often expensive and hard to find, Keville says.

Body Oils

Body oils made from herbs or essential oils are suitable for massage but can also be offered as an alternative to some internal remedies. Keville, for instance, recalls taking care of a young boy with a stomachache who refused every natural remedy in her well-stocked cupboards. He finally settled for a tummy rub with a body oil containing essential oils that aid digestion. Later, he said that it was the best medicine anyone had ever given him, and he even asked for a bottle to take home.

If you add heat-supplying herbs or essential oils such as cinnamon, cloves, or ground red pepper (cayenne) to your body oil, it becomes a liniment suitable for rubbing into sore muscles, Keville says. Body oil is also the basis for making facial creams and skin lotions. While herbal body oils are extremely versatile, they usually take longer to act than internal remedies.

Compresses

Compresses are quick to assemble yet very effective for a variety of problems—headaches, bleeding, bruises, muscle cramps, sore throats, and almost any time when alternating hot and cold is needed to increase circulation. They are also used to bolster immunity and increase lymph flow, especially when there is an internal infection or a growth, such as a fibroid, Keville says. Making a compress is easy: Soak a soft cloth in a strong herbal tea, a diluted tincture or glycerite, essential oil, or aromatic water. Wring out the cloth, then fold it and lay it on the skin. A castor-oil pack is a compress in which the cloth is soaked in warm castor oil (sometimes combined with essential oils). The soaked cloth is placed on the skin and covered with a hot-water bottle to retain heat. The one inconvenience with compresses is that to use them, you must either lie down or tie them in place.

Herbal Baths

Besides providing a relaxing and luxurious way to take your medicine, a bath can combine herbs with other therapies, including aromatherapy—the use of fragrant herbs or essential oils—and hydrotherapy, which uses alternating hot and cold water treatment to stimulate circulation. Heat relaxes the muscles, and cold reduces swelling. When you consider that stress is the most common factor in promoting disease, an herbal bath may be one of the most important herbal treatments available, Keville says. Baths are also useful in treating certain skin problems, and the steam that rises off a bath containing essential oils can be a treatment in itself for various breathing and circulation problems.

A variation on a full-body bath is a foot or hand bath, popularized by French herbalist Maurice Messegue and French aromatherapist Marguerite Maury. In his book *Of People and Plants*, Messegue reports some amazing cures for serious problems using only herbal foot and hand baths. To make a foot or hand bath, add 5 to 10 drops of essential oil or 1 cup of strong herb tea to 1 quart of water in a large basin and stir well to distribute essential oils.

Poultice

A poultice is made by pounding, blending, or even chewing a fresh plant into a sticky paste, which is then spread on an injury and sometimes wrapped with a bandage to keep it in place. Keville concedes that it may look a little strange and can be quite messy, but its effectiveness should outweigh any of your qualms.

One of Keville's friends, Gary, a carpenter, was accustomed to getting splinters while working in his wood shop, so he did not think much about a splinter in his leg last year—until he discovered that a nasty infection had developed, Keville recalls. He tried an herbal salve, but it was no match for the infection. He spent weeks trying a variety of antibiotics. The boils did heal, only to reappear persistently in different locations, sometimes opening into raw, painful sores. Gary decided to turn back to herbs, but with a different approach. He applied three poultices of fresh plantain and comfrey daily. It took a few weeks for his sores to heal completely, but he was finally free of the infection.

Another type of poultice is made from clay and/or dried, powdered herbs that are moistened into a paste using a tincture, strong herb tea, or water. Sometimes essential oils are added. Because this type of poultice comes in handy so often, Keville usually carries some with her for emergencies. Once, when attending an herb retreat, someone tapped her on the shoulder. "Quick," he said urgently. "A woman working in the dining room just got stung by a bee and she is allergic to them." When Keville reached the victim, another herbalist had already given the woman some echinacea, and someone had run to her cabin for a prescription antidote.

As Keville coated the woman's swollen hand with her poultice, the woman said, "Oh, that feels so good!" Keville nodded, preoccupied with watching for signs of a reaction. Indeed, red lines were radiating from the sting and a deep red flush was creeping up the woman's neck. Then, as quickly as they had appeared, both the red lines and the flush receded and disappeared.

Note: Anyone suffering a severe allergic reaction to a bee sting must immediately see a doctor or take medicine prescribed for the allergy.

Salve

A salve is basically a thickened herbal oil. Olive oil, which is considered healing to the skin, is the most common salve base, but other vegetable oils can also be used. To help a salve adhere to the skin, try adding beeswax, Keville suggests.

Salves are used on almost all skin problems, including minor bruises and cuts, scrapes, rashes, eczema, and swelling. Exceptions include any burn beyond a minor one (because of its oil base, a salve will hold the heat of a burn and cause more pain), the oozing stage of poison oak or poison ivy, and infected open wounds. Keville once taught a weekend herb seminar attended by a man named Juan, who clearly was paying little attention. He did, however, take home some herbal salve that the class had made. Recalling that Keville had said it was a first-aid kit in itself, he took the salve to Mexico, where he encountered other travelers with all sorts of skin problems: foot blisters, chapped lips, scrapes and cuts, infected slivers, diaper rash, a rash from an unknown plant, bruises, hemorrhoids and sunburns. He doled out small amounts of salve, and as word spread through the village, the locals began requesting his *crema herbal*. Juan returned home with an empty jar and immediately called to sign up for next year's herb seminar, promising to pay attention this time, Keville says. He learned more the second time, and to this day he says that the herbal salve is the most important item in his first-aid kit. Just about the only disadvantage of salves is that they can stain your clothes.

Homemade Medicinal and Cosmetic Herbal Products

If you are ambitious enough to make your own herbal products, these basic, generic recipes will guide you, Keville says. The general uses for these preparations are discussed earlier in this chapter. Your homemade products will cost a fraction of what the same preparations cost in the store, and you can avoid a lot of the unwanted extras, such as preservatives, stabilizers, and colorants that are found in many products sold in health food stores. Manufacturers, for instance, tend to use a lot of fixatives and preservatives because they are concerned that someone might sue them if a product is spoiled. Many herbs and most essential oils, however, contain their own natural preservatives, and beeswax is a great natural preservative.

You probably already have everything necessary to transform your kitchen into an herbal laboratory, Keville says. In cooking up herbal formulas, be sure to use glass measuring cups and pans made of stainless steel or some other nonreactive material. The proportions can change slightly according to the weight and absorbency of the herbs.

Tincture Formula

1 ounce dried or powdered herbs

About 5 ounces vodka

If using dried herbs, chop finely with a knife or in a blender. Place the chopped or powdered herbs in a clean glass jar; do not pack them tightly or the alcohol will not be able to saturate them.

Cover the herbs with just enough vodka so that they are completely submerged and can slosh around a little. (Vodka contains only alcohol and water. One hundred–proof vodka is preferable, but 80-proof vodka will do. The former is 50 percent alcohol and 50 percent water; the latter is 40 percent alcohol and 60 percent water.) If there seems to be too much or not enough vodka, adjust the amounts as necessary.

Put a tight lid on the jar and store for 2 weeks at room temperature. (A dark shelf is fine since a tincture does not need light to process.) Shake the contents once or twice a day to redistribute the herbs in the alcohol. If you are using powdered herbs, stir them with a spoon every day to keep them from clumping together.

After 2 weeks, strain out the herb pulp using a coffee filter or fine kitchen strainer. Discard the pulp. Store the liquid in a cool place; the tincture should last for 6 years or longer.

Glycerite Formula

1   ounce herbs

6   ounces glycerin

4   ounces distilled water

Chop the herbs finely with a knife or in a blender. Place in a clean glass jar; do not pack them too tightly.

In a small bowl, combine the glycerin and water; pour over the herbs in the jar. Put a tight lid on the jar. Keep at room temperature. Shake the contents every day to redistribute the herbs.

After 2 weeks, strain out the herb pulp using a coffee filter or fine kitchen strainer. Discard the pulp. Store the liquid in a cool place out of direct sunlight; the glycerite will last for at least 2 years.

Herbal Vinegar Formula

1   ounce fresh or dried herbs

About 5 ounces vinegar

Chop the herbs finely with a knife or in a blender. Place in a clean glass jar, packed loosely.

Add just enough vinegar to cover the herbs (different herbs have different levels of absorbency, so you may need more or less vinegar). Put a tight lid on the jar. Keep at room temperature.

After 2 weeks, strain out the herb pulp using a coffee filter or fine kitchen strainer. Discard the pulp. Herbal vinegars will last for years.

Herbal Syrup

6 **tablespoons herbs**

1 **pint water**

4 **ounces glycerin**

1 **ounce rice syrup or fruit syrup (or honey, for children over 2 years old)**

In a large uncovered saucepan, bring the herbs and water to a boil. Remove from the heat, cover, and steep for 30 minutes.

Using a coffee filter or fine kitchen strainer, strain the herbs from the resulting tea. Discard the herbs and return the liquid to the saucepan. Return the saucepan to heat, allow the tea to simmer, then turn off the heat. Measure out 1 cup of tea and stir in the glycerin and syrup or honey while the mixture is still warm. Let cool. Store in the refrigerator. The syrup will last for at least 6 months.

Herbal Pills

1½ **teaspoons honey**

1 **tablespoon powdered herbs**

 Extra powdered herbs

In a small saucepan over low heat, warm the honey. Add the herbs bit by bit, stirring as you go. The consistency should resemble a thick, sticky dough.

Remove from the heat. When it is cool enough to handle, roll the mixture into pea-size balls between the palms of your hands or on wax paper secured to a work surface. Let dry on the work surface for about 30 minutes, then roll in more powdered herbs so that the outside is not as sticky. This makes soft pills that can last for at least a year.

Body Oil

2 ounces dried herbs

About 1 pint vegetable oil

Chop the herbs very fine. Place in a container and pour in just enough oil to cover. (Use more or less oil as needed.) Stir to release trapped air bubbles. (Avoid using powdered herbs; they absorb oil like a sponge and clog the strainer. If powdered herbs are all you have, stir the powder every day to keep it from clumping together.)

Heat the herbs and oil for about 5 hours at approximately 80°F. You can use a double boiler on the stove top, the oven, an electric turkey cooker, or a slow cooker set on the lowest temperature. (If the setting on your appliance is not low enough, turn it on and off and monitor the temperature using a kitchen thermometer.) Or you can put the herb-oil mixture outside on a hot day; the temperature of the oil in the jar will be about 10 degrees cooler than the surrounding air. This will take 2 to 3 days, unless the air temperature is in the 90s. When done, strain out the herbs with a fine kitchen strainer, pressing out the oil with the back of a spoon. If any herb particles come through the strainer, re-strain the oil through a coffee filter. (These fine pieces can irritate skin when the oil is rubbed over it.)

Store the herb oil in a glass or plastic container in a cool place. The oil will keep for several months; stored in the refrigerator, it will keep even longer.

Body oil can be thickened by adding a natural thickener such as cocoa butter, lanolin, or beeswax and then heating the mixture slightly. For every cup of vegetable oil, add ¼ teaspoon cocoa butter, ½ to 2 teaspoons liquid lanolin, or ½ ounce (by weight) beeswax. If the consistency is not exactly what you want, reheat the mixture and add more oil or thickener.

Body oils can also be made with fresh herbs, though this takes a little more care since fresh herbs can easily spoil or become a breeding ground for mold. Herbs that contain a lot of water, such as comfrey, are better used in dried form, but some herbs, such as St.-John's-wort, are far more potent when fresh. If you use fresh herbs, follow the same directions given above for making oils from dried herbs, but be sure to use a container that is absolutely dry. The herbs should be completely submerged, all air bubbles stirred out, and the oil filled to the very top of the jar to discourage bacterial growth. If your oil begins to smell unpleasant, or if the herbs appear spotted or rotten, your oil has spoiled and shouldn't be used. Because fresh herbs contain a certain amount of water, you may have some water in the bottom of the container when you are done preparing this formula. If so, discard it after you pour the oil off the top, even if it means throwing away the last bit of oil.

Body Oil with Essential Oil

4 ounces vegetable oil

½ teaspoon essential oil

Combine the vegetable oil and essential oil. Store in a glass or plastic container in the refrigerator.

Healing Salve

1 cup Body Oil (page 43)

¾ ounce beeswax (by weight)

8 drops essential oil (optional)

Combine the Body Oil and beeswax. Heat the mixture just enough to melt the wax. Add the essential oil (if using). Stir, then pour into wide-mouthed jars. Let cool.

Store at room temperature. This salve will keep for 6 months. If you have difficulty finding beeswax, check the telephone book for a bee supply store, craft store, or beekeeper and ask for pure beeswax.

Herbal Compress

5 drops essential oil

Small bowl of lukewarm water

Add the essential oil to the water. Soak a soft cloth in the mixture and wring it out. Fold the cloth and apply to the afflicted area.

Skin-Healing Poultice

1 handful herbs

4 ounces water

Combine the herbs and water in a blender. Process into a thick slurry. Spread on the wound, holding the poultice in place by wrapping gauze around it. Leave the poultice on the wound for 20 minutes to 1 hour.

To store for future emergencies, freeze the poultice in ice-cube trays. Keep the cubes in a plastic bag or freezer container. When you need a poultice, thaw out a cube in a pan at room temperature.

Herbal Safeguards

Herbal medicine is generally safer than conventional medicine. But you need to understand what can go wrong and how to protect yourself.

Herbal remedies. They're natural. Heck, they're from plants. No synthetics. No muss. No fuss. They have to be safe, right? Too bad it's not that simple.

While lots of natural cures are extremely effective and helpful, folks tend to forget one crucial point: Herbal remedies are medicine, which means that they pack some serious power—and the potential to do harm.

Even an experienced herbalist can make mistakes, says Varro E. Tyler, Ph.D., Sc.D., former professor of pharmacognosy at Purdue University in West Lafayette, Indiana, and author of *The New Honest Herbal* and *Herbs of Choice*. After all, there are some 300,000 higher plant species that are all chemically distinct. Yet a really good herbalist might know 1,000 to 2,000 species. And new information about herbs is coming to light every day. In fact, studies show that a few herbs long considered safe for internal use are actually hazardous. Large doses of comfrey, for instance, a traditional digestive remedy, are now known to cause liver damage. What's more, any herb—like food—can cause an allergic reaction in some people. So you have to exercise some caution.

For healthy individuals who are not pregnant, the herbs in this book are all considered safe in recommended amounts. However, pregnant women should consult their obstetricians before using any medicinal

Herbs to Shun while Pregnant

As a general rule, you shouldn't take herbs while you're pregnant unless you discuss your selections with your obstetrician.

There's a good reason for this. Quite a few herbs can increase the risk of miscarriage. Maine herbalist Deb Soule, author of the feminist herbal *The Roots of Healing*, advises pregnant women to avoid the following herbs: barberry root bark, cascara sagrada, feverfew, juniper berries, mugwort, pennyroyal, pokeroot, rue, senna, southernwood, tansy, thuja, and wormwood.

Be wary of balsam pear, chervil, Chinese angelica, evening primrose, hernandia, hyptis, mayapple, mountain mint, and St.-John's-wort, too, suggests James A. Duke, Ph.D., a retired U.S. Department of Agriculture botanist and author of *The Green Pharmacy*.

You should limit your consumption of caffeine as well. One study showed what the researchers called a "strong association of caffeine intake during pregnancy and fetal loss." As little as 163 milligrams of caffeine per day—the amount in one to two cups of brewed coffee—might double the risk of spontaneous abortion.

In addition, here are a few more don'ts during pregnancy: Don't smoke, don't drink alcohol, and again, don't take any drugs, including over-the-counter products, except on the advice of your obstetrician.

herbs (or pharmaceuticals). Most herbal medicines should not be given to children under age 2. Children under 16 and anyone over 65 should dilute herbal preparations to reduce the dose. And those with chronic medical conditions should consult their physicians before supplementing medical therapies with herbs. Here are a few other strategies that you can use to protect yourself.

Be knowledgeable, not gullible. Medicinal herbs are available at health food stores, herb shops, supplement outlets, some pharmacies and supermarkets, and through mail-order catalogs. They're marketed in so many different forms that many people become confused.

The savvy consumer needs to be open-minded to new, improved methods of extracting and preparing herbs but wary of sales pitches that promote one product over another. One of the best ways to sort through this marketing confusion is to educate yourself and seek out a store with knowledgeable clerks. Herbs are wondrous healers, but be realistic about their abilities, says Kathi Keville, director of the American Herb Association and author of *Herbs for Health and Healing*.

Determining a reliable producer can often be tricky. It may take some trial and error before you find a producer whose product you can put your trust in, Dr. Tyler says.

Read labels carefully. Check that both the quantity of the extract per dose and the concentration of one or more active ingredients is stated. Compare the recommended dosage with that found in Dr. Tyler's book *Herbs of Choice* or other scientific herbal literature.

Get the right stuff. Unless you are sure of an herb's identity, don't take it, advises James A. Duke, Ph.D., a retired U.S. Department of Agriculture botanist and author of *The Green Pharmacy.* This rule applies mainly to people who are picking herbs in the wild, of course. People have been known to eat poisonous or dangerous plants simply because they misidentified an herb and took something other than what they thought they were taking. The classic killer is poison hemlock, which looks rather like wild parsley or wild parsnip.

Whatever herb you're taking, learn as much as you can about what to expect from it. If anything unexpected happens, stop taking whatever it is and check with an expert you trust.

Don't play doctor. Herbal devotees sometimes get the idea that they can diagnose illness and come up with herbs to treat it. But diagnosis is a separate art, and one best left to physicians, Dr. Duke says.

Diagnosing illness is not easy, and sometimes even good doctors make mistakes. But physicians' diagnostic batting average is usually better than that of anyone who has not had medical training. Once you're confident of a diagnosis, then you can discuss with your physician how to treat it: drugs, herbs, some combination of the two, or changes in diet, exercise, or lifestyle.

Listen to your body. All medicines—natural or synthetic—have side effects, Dr. Duke says. That's why you have to watch yourself when taking any new herb for the first time.

If you have an unpleasant reaction to an herb, such as dizziness, nausea, or headache, cut back on your dosage or stop taking the herb. If the herb doesn't feel right, don't take it, Dr. Duke says.

Itch and scratch mean stop. People can be allergic to anything. Even if you have no known allergies, you might be allergic to a new herb you try. Be careful. Listen to your body. If you develop any unusual symptoms, stop taking your new herb and consult an allergist or physician, Dr. Duke says.

If you develop any difficulty breathing within 30 minutes or so of trying a new herb, food, or drug, call 911 immediately. You may be having an anaphylactic reaction, the most severe form of allergic reaction. Anaphylactic reactions can prove rapidly fatal unless treated promptly.

Anaphylactic reactions to herbs are rare. Just be careful and understand the possible risks.

Some herbs don't get along. Pharmaceutical medicines sometimes interact badly with each other and with certain foods. The same goes for herbal medicines, only many herbal reference books neglect to mention this, Dr. Duke warns. Always be particularly careful when taking more than one drug or herb or combination of drug and herb. Bad interactions are always possible. If you suspect a bad interaction, consult your physician or pharmacist.

In particular, beware of the class of antidepressants known as monoamine oxidase (MAO) inhibitors. These drugs can interact badly with wine, cheese, and many other foods. If you take a pharmaceutical MAO inhibitor, you shouldn't eat these foods, Dr. Duke says.

The antidepressant herb, St.-John's-wort, is also an MAO inhibitor, so the same food restrictions apply. If you take St.-John's-wort regularly, consult a physician, pharmacist, or consumer drug guide about foods to avoid.

Blaze one trail at a time. Too many people listen to both their physicians and their herbalists and do what both advise. Usually, there's no problem with this—for example, when a physician gives you sleeping pills for insomnia and an herbalist recommends a hot bath before bed with a blend of sedative aromatherapy oils.

But just as too many cooks can spoil the broth, too many health practitioners can also be too much of a good thing. Let's say that your physician prescribes an MAO inhibitor for depression and your herbalist recommends St.-John's-wort, also an MAO inhibitor. Then you may wind up taking too much, Dr. Duke says. Or let's say that your physician prescribes half an aspirin a day to prevent heart attack, and your herbalist tells you to drink a cup of willow bark or wintergreen tea a day. The teas contain the herbal equivalent of aspirin, and you might wind up taking more than you need with more anti-clotting action than you want.

To avoid the too-many-cooks problem, be sure to tell your physician and your herbalist about all the medicines that you're taking as well as any unusual foods that you might be eating, Dr. Duke says. And if you're consulting an herbalist, be sure that he's also informed of any other medications that you're taking.

Meet the Pasha of Plants

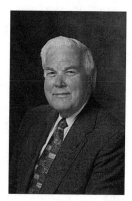

Varro E. Tyler, Ph.D., Sc.D., former professor of pharmacognosy at Purdue University in West Lafayette, Indiana, author of The New Honest Herbal *and* Herbs of Choice, *and* Prevention *magazine columnist, is one of the nation's foremost experts on natural healing. He believes in the promise of herbal cures.*

To someone like Dr. Tyler, raw nature is the original drugstore. Aspirin came from willow bark; digitalis for the heart came from common foxglove.

"Plant drugs make up conventional medicine in two-thirds of the world. But in this country it's still classified as unconventional medicine," says Dr. Tyler.

Why?

In America herbal medicine got a bad name during the first half of this century, when elixirs, pills, and potions claimed to cure anything that ailed you. Today, herbal medicines may not have this creative labeling, but testimonials for herbal remedies still tend toward the mystical or folkloric. Literature on the subject is often inaccurate; herbal claims are often outrageous, Dr. Tyler says. "Paraherbalism" is the term he uses to describe the suspect branch of plant medicine that operates without a scientific net.

"Only 20 percent—maybe less—of the claims made for herbal medicinals in this country are valid," he says. "I want to see clinical studies—data, evidence—that an herbal product does what it says it does."

So Dr. Tyler has devoted much of his life to correcting errant herbalism and constructing what he calls rational herbalism. To that end, he has written two comprehensive books to guide both professionals and consumers through the overwhelming phytomedicinal maze of the modern health food market: *The New Honest Herbal* and *Herbs of Choice*. He has also written scientific textbooks, including the standard text *Pharmacognosy*, for which he was senior author. In all, Dr. Tyler has written 18 books, either in whole or in part, plus more than 270 scientific articles.

He has been honored almost from the beginning of his career. Right after college, he spent a year as an Eli Lilly Research Fellow, studying plant science at Yale University. In 1966, he won the American Pharmaceutical Association Foundation Research Achievement Award in natural products for his work on the rye fungus (and migraine medicine) ergot. In 1996, Dr. Tyler was named Economic Botanist of the Year. In between there were many more accolades and awards.

The Mysteries of the Apothecary

How did the 6-foot-tall scientist grow up to be the Hippocrates of herbs? One reason was his hometown, a small riverbank farming community in Nebraska called Nebraska City. Even though it contained only 7,000 people, it supported five drugstores. Pharmacies punctuated Dr. Tyler's everyday environment.

"I started to work in a pharmacy behind the soda fountain when I was 12. The boss was a very congenial man who wanted to show all the boys who worked for him some of the mysteries of the apothecary. So we would fill things like cold capsules and influenza capsules. Everything had to be powdered and mixed and encapsulated by hand. That really got me kind of interested in pharmacy."

Even his first name, which came to him by way of his country-doctor grandfather, has a medicinal ring to it. "Varro was a Roman encyclopedist often credited with having invented the germ theory. Long before microscopes, he thought that disease was caused by little animalcules that infected people," Dr. Tyler says.

So if Varro Tyler hadn't gone into pharmaceutical studies, it would have been a surprise. But he accepted the nudge of fate, graduated from the University of Nebraska in 1949, and followed an inspiring pharmacognosy professor to the University of Connecticut, where he earned both master's and doctorate degrees. After school he taught for a while at the University of Nebraska. Then he went out to the University of Washington in Seattle, where he fell in love with fungi, both to research and to eat. With fellow mycologists he stalked the Northwest forests, gathering chanterelles to cook into feasts. He also investigated the ergot that got him honored. "And ergot is still used for everything from migraine headaches to controlling postpartum hemorrhage," he says.

After Seattle Dr. Tyler went to Purdue University, where he continued his herbal career and served as professor of pharmacognosy and dean of the schools of pharmacy, nursing, and health sciences. He also served as vice president of academic affairs. Just before he retired, he introduced a new course for his college students called Drugs from Nature.

Despite his achievements, honors, and travels, Dr. Tyler still has one burning ambition. "I'd like to convince people that herbal medicine can be put on a useful scientific and clinical basis. I'd like to get it away from all the hype and hyperbole.

"I personally am convinced that so many of these plants can be very useful products—milder and less expensive than many of the drugs we have now. My ambition—the goal toward which I'd still like to work—is to see sensible regulations, properly implemented, that would control herbal drugs in this country," Dr. Tyler says. "To go into a health food store to buy a product and not find on the label what a supplement is good for—what effects and side effects to expect—is wrong."

Straight Talk from the Honest Herbalist

Varro E. Tyler, Ph.D., Sc.D., former professor of pharmacognosy at Purdue University in West Lafayette, Indiana, author of The New Honest Herbal *and* Herbs of Choice, Prevention *magazine columnist, and America's foremost expert on plant-derived medicine, answers your questions about using herbs to treat colds and flu, PMS, arthritis, high blood pressure, and other ailments.*

Q: I've read several conflicting reports on how long to take echinacea. One says to not use it on a continuing basis, while another indicates that you should take it for 14 days but gives no further information. I was advised to take it for three weeks, then stop for a week to prevent it from losing its effectiveness. I am really confused; can you help?

A: I hope so. The German Commission E, considered the worldwide authority on herbal medicine, recommends that echinacea should not be used either internally or externally for longer than eight successive weeks. Specialists had always presumed that this was based on evidence that the herb lost its effectiveness after that length of time.

At the American Chemical Society in 1996, professor Dr. H. Schilcher, longtime member of the commission, was asked the reason for this time limitation. He replied that there were no specific studies indicating loss of effectiveness or of toxicity following continued consumption. Rather, the members of Commission E had imposed this restriction based on general safety and efficacy. In other words, if echinacea hadn't worked for whatever condition it was being taken for at the end of eight weeks, there was no reason to continue using it.

As a pharmacist who doesn't believe in taking drugs if you don't need them, I agree with this conclusion. In fact, since echinacea is mostly used for colds or flu, I would recommend that if it has not helped relieve symptoms in two or, at the most, three weeks, stop taking it. Echinacea is most effective when taken at the first sign of sniffles or scratchy throat. If you choose to take echinacea longer, it probably won't hurt you, but it probably won't do much good, either.

Q: Every now and then, my arthritis flares up and is really quite painful. Aspirin upsets my stomach, so a friend recommended alfalfa pills. Should I try them?

A: Alfalfa has a reputation in folk medicine as being useful for treating rheumatism and arthritis. This use dates back to the very early years of this century. Unfortunately, in all the intervening years, no one has ever proved that alfalfa was good for anything, except nourishing livestock. Because it is such a popular animal fodder, the chemical composition of alfalfa has been extensively studied, but clinical trials of its effectiveness on various medical conditions are simply nonexistent. Therefore, I see no reason to use alfalfa pills.

There is also no evidence that alfalfa seeds or sprouts, often used in salads, would be beneficial either.

Q: Is chaparral safe? I've heard that it causes some liver problems, but it's still available.

A: Chaparral, or creosote bush, is very common in the dry lands of the southwestern United States. For more than 25 years, the herb enjoyed an underground reputation as a cancer cure, but its effectiveness was never proven scientifically. But neither were any adverse effects reported.

Then, in 1992, four cases of liver toxicity associated with chaparral consumption became known. One was so serious that the patient required a liver transplant. This prompted the Food and Drug Administration (FDA) Center for Food Safety and Applied Nutrition to caution consumers not to use chaparral. The various herb trade associations also asked their members not to sell the herb.

Subsequently, the American Herbal Products Association (AHPA) employed university medical experts to review the four cases. They concluded that the toxicity was idiosyncratic and that there was no evidence to indicate that chaparral was toxic. In April 1995, the AHPA gave the green light to its members to sell chaparral once again. The other major trade associations refused to reverse their sales ban.

Here the matter stands today. The FDA warning against the use of chaparral is still in effect. Certainly, persons with known liver disease would be at considerable risk taking it. Besides, until chaparral has been shown to be good for something, there is really no reason to do so.

Q: I have read that ground red pepper (cayenne) consumption can lower blood pressure. Is that a fact?

A: Cayenne pepper, the fruit of several species of capsicum, contains varying amounts of the pungent chemical capsaicin. Externally, capsaicin (an over-the-counter drug) is applied in a cream or gel base to relieve intractable pain caused by conditions ranging from arthritic joints to migraine to shingles. Such usage is approved by the FDA.

Caution: Avoid getting the product in your eyes and tender parts of your skin; it will burn.

When eaten or drunk as a tea, red pepper stimulates secretions, so it may help relieve nasal stuffiness associated with colds. According to folklore, it also has been used to aid digestion and help expel gas that causes a bloated feeling. Up to ½ teaspoon is the recommended dose, depending on the content of capsaicin and your sensitivity. Start with smaller amounts to see how much your mouth can tolerate.

Versatile as it may be, red pepper has no proven effect on blood pressure. This fiction was popularized in the 1970s by an herbalist who claimed that it helped the blood vessels regain elasticity, thus normalizing blood pressure. Unfortunately, such an effect has never been demonstrated, but the myth lingers on.

Q: I read an article claiming that wild yam is a source of sex hormones. Then I got an advertisement for a wild-yam cream that says that it relieves the symptoms of premenstrual syndrome (PMS), menopause, and osteoporosis in women and helps treat male-pattern baldness by increasing testosterone levels. How does this miracle herb work?

A: It doesn't—at least pills or creams made from pure wild yam don't. This kind of advertising hype is made possible by the common misconception that because certain compounds contained in the wild yam (steroidal precursors) can be converted to various hormones in the chemical laboratory, they also make the same conversion in the body. That is not the case. The human body and the chemical lab are two very different things. However, promoters use this confusion to support their far-fetched claims.

If wild-yam creams or pills have any progestin activity, it is because the hormone progesterone or a related chemical with similar activity has been added to them. This is known in the trade as spiking. Read the ads for such products closely. You will see that they are very carefully worded so as not to rule out that possibility.

A similar situation exists with sarsaparilla. This root of various species of *Smilax* is being incorporated into a number of preparations intended either to relieve PMS and menopausal symptoms or, more commonly, to enhance athletic performance and help build muscles. It's often billed as a "natural testosterone source." This, too, is based on the belief that natural steroids, sarsapogenin and smilagenin, in the plant are converted into androgens or estrogens in the human body. Not so.

Q: A recent article in a medical journal noted that Siberian ginseng contains glycosides chemically similar to those in digitalis and that consumption of the herb causes increased levels of digoxin in a patient's blood. Does this mean that it is unsafe for persons on digitalis to take Siberian ginseng?

A: The article that you quote was apparently based on two false premises. Siberian ginseng—better called eleuthero, to avoid confusion with real ginseng—does not contain glycosides that are similar chemically or in their effects to those of digitalis. Eleuthero, derived from *Eleutherococcus senticosus*, is, however, often adulterated with another plant known as Chinese silk vine. This occurs frequently because the Chinese names of the two plants are similar.

Chinese silk vine contains a number of cardiac glycosides very similar to those of digitalis. The findings that you note were almost certainly due to that herb, not to eleuthero. Unless Siberian ginseng can be certified to be pure and not contaminated by Chinese silk vine, it shouldn't be used by patients taking digitalis glycosides. Medical authorities do warn against consuming eleuthero if you have high blood pressure.

Q: Capsules containing standardized *Ginkgo biloba* extract are relatively expensive. Why can't I collect the leaves from the ginkgo tree that's growing in my yard and make them into a tea with the same beneficial properties as the capsules?

A: The extract found in *Ginkgo biloba* capsules is highly concentrated to a standard of 24 percent of flavonoid glycosides and 6 percent ginkgolides. This represents an average 50-fold concentration of the constituents in the leaf. Assuming that the active constituents were completely extracted in a tea (an unrealistic expectation), this would require consumption of tea made from as much as 10 grams of leaf material daily—also an unrealistic expectation.

But that is not the biggest problem. In its natural state, ginkgo leaf contains anacardic and ginkgolic acids, both highly allergenic. These compounds are closely related chemically to urushiol, the active toxin in poison ivy, and produce about the same effect. They are removed from the concentrated ginkgo extract, but they would be present in tea made from the unprocessed leaf. So these allergens also prevent you from using ginkgo leaf tea as an effective remedy.

Q: I heard a rumor that St.-John's-wort, widely used to treat depression, can cause liver problems. What's the scoop?

A: There is no scientific evidence or clinical evidence supporting the assertion that consumption of normal therapeutic amounts of St.-John's-wort causes liver toxicity.

In a study of 3,250 people taking a concentrated extract of the herb three times daily for four weeks, the most common side effects—each reported in fewer than 20 people—were gastrointestinal symptoms, allergic reactions, and fatigue. Notably absent from the list of adverse reactions was any report of liver toxicity.

The rumor about liver problems with St.-John's-wort may stem from the use of large quantities of the herb, along with high doses of other drugs, for its potential anti–HIV activity. Such cases would certainly not be typical of normal therapeutic use of the herb for its antidepressant effect.

Q: I was told that powdered stevia leaves, a noncaloric artificial sweetener, have never been approved by the FDA. Is it safe to sweeten my tea with stevia?

A: Stevia, the leaves of *Stevia rebaudiana*, has been used by Guarani Indians in Paraguay for hundreds of years to sweeten their bitter maté, a kind of tea. The main active constituent, a glycoside known as stevioside, is about 200 to 300 times as sweet as ordinary sugar and contains practically no calories.

Stevioside is now widely used in South Korea, Japan, and Taiwan for sweetening everything from pickles to dried fish to ice cream. No adverse effects have been reported in these countries.

In the United States, stevia is sold as a dietary supplement under the Dietary Supplement Health and Education Act, but technically, the FDA has never approved the product. In fact, the FDA actually embargoed the importation of stevia from 1991 to 1995 on the basis of a lack of proven safety, a questionable decision.

In my view of the extensive studies of stevia—including long-term toxicity trials—conducted in Japan, I believe that it's all right to use it to sweeten your tea. Stevia is available in health food stores. A ¼- to ½-teaspoon serving per cup should do the trick. Start small; you can always add more.

Q: I have heard conflicting stories about catnip. One claims that the tea is an effective sleep aid. The other says that it causes hallucinations. Which is correct?

A: Tea prepared from the catnip plant has an ancient reputation as a sleep promoter and nerve tonic. Its effectiveness has not been confirmed by clinical trials in humans. It has been shown to induce sleep in young chickens in low doses. At very high doses, however, sleep was impaired.

The assertion that catnip has psychedelic properties arose from a classic gaffe in medical literature. In 1969, the *Journal of the American Medical Association* published a paper authored by two physicians noting that patients who smoked catnip experienced effects very similar to those produced by marijuana. The authors illustrated both plants, but the drawing of catnip was mislabeled *Cannabis sativa* and that of marijuana was mislabeled *Nepeta cataria*. More than 1,600 letters to the editors pointed out that is was little wonder that the smokers became intoxicated because they were indeed smoking marijuana, not catnip.

So not to worry: Catnip will not make you high.

Catnip tea appears to be quite safe if drunk in reasonable amounts—no more than 2 to 3 cups daily. One famous herbalist even recommended it for pacifying babies. I disagree with that suggestion because I don't believe in giving any herbs to young children. After all, most herbs are not approved drugs, and long-term safety studies are often lacking. Youngsters are sometimes more susceptible to the effects of medications than adults. No absolute method exists for calculating the proper dose for an infant or a child. If knowledgeable adults want to take them, that's different.

Incidentally, both catnip and another sedative herb, valerian, stimulate cats but tranquilize people. How's that for irony?

part 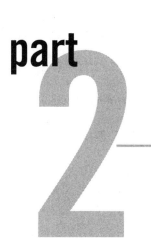 **2**

The Herbal Pharmacy

Natural Prescriptions

for Healing

What Can Cure You?

A quick head-to-toe user's guide to the best herbal remedies for each part of your body.

Mental relaxation: Hops, lavender, passionflower, St.-John's-wort, valerian

Mental stimulation: Maté

Fever: Meadowsweet, white willow, witch hazel, yarrow

Headache/migraine: Chamomile, feverfew, ginger, ginkgo, white willow

Sore throat/cough: Blueberry, chamomile, goldenseal, marsh mallow, rose, sage, St.-John's-wort, slippery elm, thyme, witch hazel

Colds: Anise, echinacea, fennel, ginseng, peppermint, sage, thyme, witch hazel, yarrow

Heart: Garlic, ginseng, ginkgo, hawthorn

Nausea: Cardamom, ginger, meadowsweet

Upset stomach/indigestion: Angelica, anise, bog bean, cardamom, chamomile, cinnamon, dandelion, dill, fennel, ginger, juniper, lavender, marsh mallow, meadowsweet, peppermint, rosemary, slippery elm, thyme, yarrow

Constipation: Cascara sagrada, myrrh, senna

Diarrhea: Blueberry, goldenseal, peppermint

Hemorrhoids: Poplar, witch hazel

Urinary tract: Juniper, saw palmetto (men only), stinging nettle, uva ursi

Uterine cramps/PMS: Black cohosh, cinnamon (bloating), rosemary, witch hazel, yarrow

Muscle pain: Arnica, chamomile, paprika, St.-John's-wort, white mustard, white willow, witch hazel

Wounds/skin injuries/sunburn: Aloe, arnica, calendula, chamomile, comfrey, echinacea, goldenseal, marsh mallow, myrrh, peppermint, poplar, St.-John's-wort, slippery elm, thyme, witch hazel

Inflammation/swelling: Arnica, chamomile, juniper, marsh mallow, myrrh, St.-John's-wort, stinging nettle, white mustard

50 Powerful Herbal Cures

*Nature provides us with a mind-boggling array of herbs
to treat everything from insomnia to indigestion.
Choosing the right one for you starts here.*

Trying to keep track of all the important healing herbs probably feels a lot like those days long ago in high school when you were forced to memorize the periodic table of the elements. Information overload. Strange-sounding, and at times, unpronounceable words. The fear of getting calendula mixed up with cascara.

At least that's how many people unfamiliar with herbal treatments feel. So to help you out, here's a compilation of all the vital stuff that you need to know about these important healing herbs—trivia, uses, dosages, contraindications—in this chapter. When you want to know if it's okay to apply comfrey to a minor cut, this is the place to come.

The herbal dosages recommended in this chapter and elsewhere in the book represent a compilation of wisdom gathered from both traditional herbalists and modern scientific sources, such as Germany's Commission E. Since it was formed in the 1970s, the commission, a group of scientists appointed by Germany's equivalent of the Food and Drug Administration, has evaluated the safety and effectiveness of some 300 herbal remedies.

Of those, the commission has deemed about 200 as safe and effective for various conditions, says Varro E. Tyler, Ph.D., Sc.D., former professor of pharmacognosy at Purdue University in West Lafayette, Indiana, and author of *The New Honest Herbal* and *Herbs of Choice*.

Then, various sources whittled that list down to 50 common, safe, and effective herbs. Before using these herbs, experts suggest consulting your doctor. They also strongly recommend that pregnant or lactating women take herbal remedies with extreme caution, and that children under 2 never take herbal remedies. Children under 16 and anyone over 65 should dilute herbal preparations to reduce the dose. (For other precautions, see Herbal Safeguards, on page 45). Keeping all of these caveats in mind, here are those herbs, the conditions they may relieve, and directions for their use.

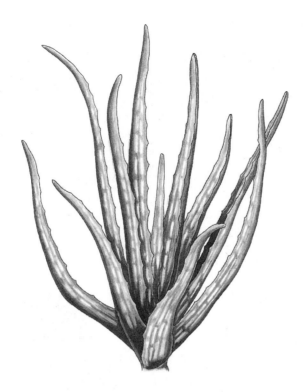

Aloe Vera (*Aloe barbadensis*)

Lore: Aloe vera was rumored to be one of Cleopatra's secret beauty ingredients.

Claims to fame: This plant may look spiky and rough, but it's a softy inside. In fact, the clear gel within aloe's spiny leaves can promote new skin growth, soften skin, and help heal minor cuts and burns (including sunburn) while preventing infection.

How to use: First, wash your skin with soap and water. Then, snip off a leaf of a live aloe plant, slit it open, and squeeze its healing gel onto the affected area. The gel will dry into a natural bandage that promotes healing and keeps bacteria at bay. You can also puree enough aloe leaves in a blender to make ¼ cup of puree. Make sure you peel the leaves first. Then stir in some vitamin C powder to preserve the gel. You can store it in the refrigerator—it will keep for one to two weeks—until you need it.

Cautions and recommendations: Aloe gel is safe for external use. If your skin shows signs of redness or irritation after applying aloe, discontinue use. Also, don't apply aloe to deep cuts that contain debris or won't stop bleeding. See your doctor instead.

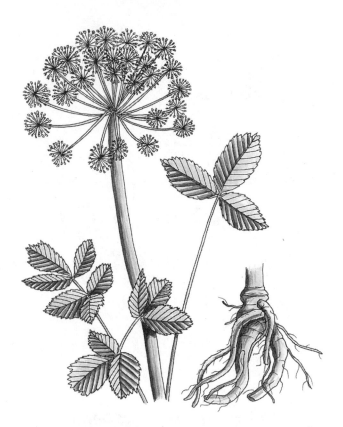

Angelica (*Angelica archangelica*)

Lore: In the seventeenth century, angelica root was used in aromatic remedies for the Black Plague.

Claims to fame: Dried angelica root can settle your upset stomach as well as stimulate your appetite.

How to use: To make a concentrated extract, use 1 teaspoon of powdered root per cup of water. Bring the mixture to a boil and simmer for 2 minutes. Then remove the mixture from the heat and let it stand for 15 minutes. Drink up to 2 cups a day. (Keep in mind, this will taste bitter.) Or you can buy a commercial extract and follow the package directions.

Cautions and recommendations: This herb is not suitable for young children. Also, be careful when outdoors. The herb can cause sun sensitivity. It has also been known to increase menstrual flow.

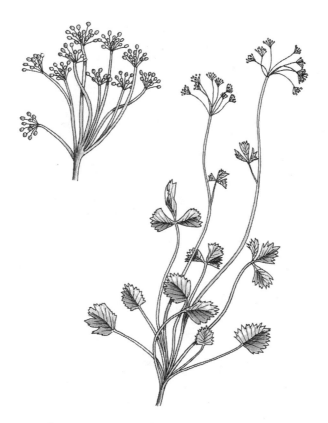

Anise (*Pimpinella anisum*)

Lore: The Roman naturalist Pliny recommended chewing fresh anise seed as a breath freshener and digestive aid after big meals.

Claims to fame: Just like some people confuse salt for a spice, many people often confuse anise with fennel. They are two separate herbs. When taken orally, dried anise seeds can calm an upset stomach, relieve gas, and help bring up phlegm from a chest cold.

How to use: To make a tea, gently crush 1 teaspoon of anise seeds per cup of boiling water. Let the mixture steep for 10 to 20 minutes and then strain before drinking. Drink up to 3 cups daily.

Cautions and recommendations: You should only ingest dried anise. The essential oil of anise is toxic and should never be taken internally. And if dried anise causes minor discomforts, such as stomach upset or diarrhea, discontinue or cut back on use.

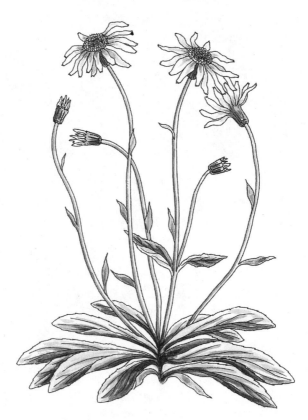

Arnica (*Arnica montana*)

Lore: Native Americans and early Europeans both made healing ointments and tinctures with arnica flowers to help relax stiff muscles and treat wounds.

Claims to fame: When applied to the skin, arnica can reduce swelling and relieve the pain of bumps and bruises.

How to use: You can buy arnica cream or salves, usually available at vitamin and health food stores. Salves should have at least 20 to 25 percent tincture. Creams should have at least 15 percent arnica oil. Follow the package directions.

Cautions and recommendations: Arnica is fairly safe when used on unbroken skin. Some people may develop a skin irritation after repeated use. If you experience irritation, discontinue use. Don't use arnica on an open wound or ingest it. Taken this way, arnica can irritate the kidneys, elevate blood pressure, and cause dizziness.

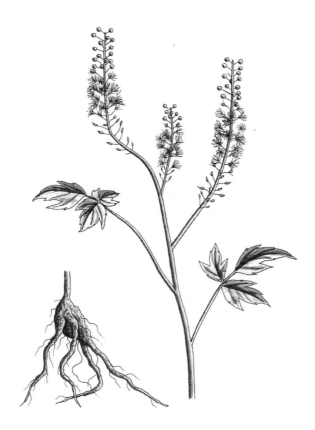

Black Cohosh (*Cimicifuga racemosa*)

Lore: At times, black cohosh has been promoted as a "hormone" herb because of its extensive use to treat women.

Claims to fame: Like soy products, black cohosh may have phyto-estrogen-like chemicals that can ease menopause, premenstrual anxiety and mood swings, and menstrual pain.

How to use: To make tea, boil ½ teaspoon of powdered root per cup of water for 30 minutes. Then let it cool. The tea will have an unpleasant aroma and bitter taste. Add lemon and honey or mix with a flavored tea. If you buy a more concentrated tincture from a store, take ½ to 1 teaspoon per day.

Cautions and recommendations: The herb can bring on an upset stomach and cause high blood pressure. Don't take black cohosh if you think that you are pregnant or if you have a heart condition. Also, be careful not to take more than the recommended amount. An overdose can cause dizziness, earache, diarrhea, or visual dimness and can affect your heart rate.

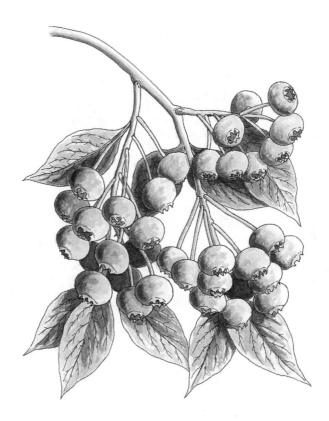

Blueberry (*Vaccinium* species)

Lore: Dried blueberries have an unbelievable shelf life. An archaeological dig in Pennsylvania once uncovered Native American clay pots that contained dried blueberries, thought to be 200 years old.

Claims to fame: Eating dried blueberries has been known to put an end to diarrhea as well as soothe sore throats.

How to use: You can chew and swallow 3 tablespoons of dried blueberries. Or you can make a tea by boiling the crushed, dried fruit in water for 10 minutes, straining, and then drinking.

Cautions and recommendations: While there are no side effects to eating blueberries, some herbalists caution against using blueberry leaves in herbal preparations because a small percentage of people can have toxic reactions.

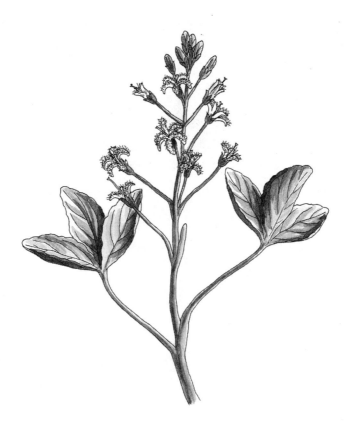

Bog Bean (*Menyanthes trifoliata*)

Lore: Native Americans would boil the roots of this bitter herb to make a strong tea medicine to treat spitting up blood and other internal problems.

Claims to fame: Bog bean, also known as buck bean, is used for treating rheumatoid arthritis. It can also speed up a sluggish digestive system as well as soothe indigestion and problems of the liver and gallbladder.

How to use: Bog bean is difficult to find in the United States. You may find commercially prepared tinctures or pills, and you should follow the package directions for these products. If you come across the dried herb, you can make an herbal tea by mixing a cup of boiling water with 1 to 2 teaspoons of the dried herb and steeping for 10 to 15 minutes. Drink up to 3 cups per day.

Cautions and recommendations: Do not use if you have colitis, and discontinue use if you develop diarrhea.

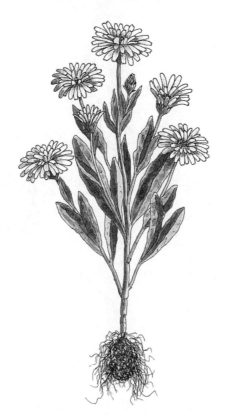

Calendula (*Calendula officinalis*)

Lore: During the Civil War, doctors on the battlefield used calendula (marigold) leaves to treat open wounds.

Claims to fame: Calendula reputedly contains natural antifungal agents that make it a perfect first-aid treatment on wounds and burns. The herb has also been used on bruises and sprains.

How to use: You can make a tea by mixing a cup of boiling water with 1 teaspoon of the petals. Let the mixture cool for 10 to 15 minutes, then soak the inflamed skin in it. You can also make a calendula compress with the cooled mixture. Or you can buy a premade cream or salve from a pharmacy or health food store and follow package directions.

Cautions and recommendations: If you have hay fever, however, you might want to avoid taking this herb, because people who are allergic to ragweed might react to calendula as well. If you take it and have a reaction—itching or any other discomfort—discontinue use.

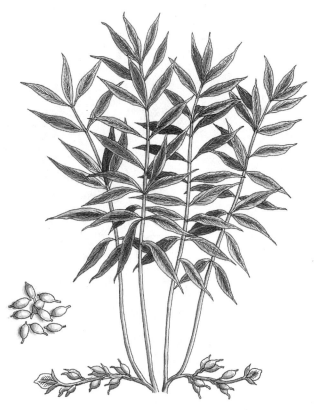

Cardamom (*Elettaria cardamomum*)

Lore: Native to East India, cardamom is a key ingredient in some varieties of curry powder. It's also used in Scandinavian pastries.

Claims to fame: These seeds can cool down the burning and nausea from indigestion.

How to use: You can make a tea by mixing ½ to 1 teaspoon of freshly crushed seeds with a cup of boiling water. Let it sit for 10 to 15 minutes before drinking. Have 3 cups a day.

Cautions and recommendations: Since heartburn and nausea can also be associated with gallstones, consult your doctor if these symptoms continue.

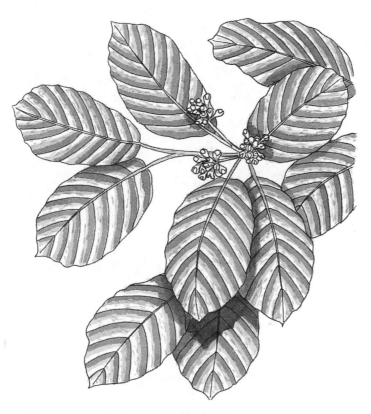

Cascara Sagrada (*Rhamnus purshiana*)

Lore: Now one of the world's most used natural laxatives, cascara didn't come into widespread use until the 1870s.

Claims to fame: The bark of this American Northwest tree can help keep you regular.

How to use: Usually, ½ teaspoon of the herb mixed with 2 cups of water will do the job. If you buy a premade concoction at a health food store or pharmacy, follow the package directions. It takes the herb about 8 hours to kick in, so be patient. Some people may have to redose after 8 hours for this laxative to work.

Cautions and recommendations: Only use cascara sagrada occasionally. If you continually use the herb, it can interfere with various types of medications, such as diurectics, heart pills, and steroids. Using the herb for great lengths of time can throw your gastrointestinal tract into a haywire mode. Avoid cascara if you have any of the following complications: intestinal problems, colitis, ulcers, or abdominal pain. Also, do not give cascara to a child younger than age 12.

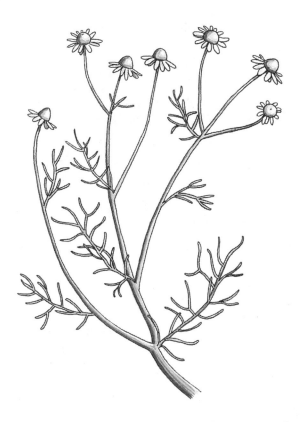

Chamomile (*Chamomilla recutita*)

Lore: Ancient Egyptians dedicated chamomile to the sun and even worshipped its powers.

Claims to fame: Studies have found that it relieves indigestion—a good reason to drink a cup after a big meal—and headaches. When used on the skin, mouth, or gums, its flowers are thought to ease bacterial infections. It can also be inhaled for inflammations and irritations of the respiratory system. Used in baths, chamomile soothes anal and genital swelling. And when rubbed into bruises or sore muscles, this herb combats swelling and relieves pain.

How to use: To make a tea, add 2 to 3 teaspoons of dried or fresh flowers to 1 cup of boiling water. Steep for 10 to 20 minutes. Drink up to 3 cups a day. Or, apply the cooled tea to the skin or gargle with it to soothe inflamed mucous membranes of the throat and mouth. For a chamomile bath, add about ¼ cup of dried flowers to the tub water, using a cloth bag.

Cautions and recommendations: Chamomile is a cousin of ragweed, and if you are allergic to one, you may be allergic to the other.

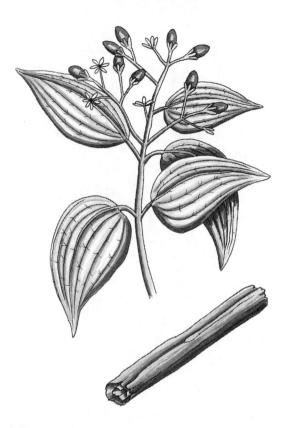

Cinnamon (*Cinnamomum verum* and *C. zeylanicum*)

Lore: Ancient Chinese herbals mention cinnamon as early as 2700 B.C. as a treatment for fever, diarrhea, and menstrual problems.

Claims to fame: You probably didn't realize that you were sprinkling dried tree bark on your oatmeal all these years. Other than tasting pretty darn good, cinnamon also can soothe away bellyache, indigestion, flatulence, and bloating.

How to use: For a warm, sweet, spicy infusion, use ½ to ¾ teaspoon of powdered herb per cup of boiling water. Drink up to 3 cups per day.

Cautions and recommendations: Though the spice can be sprinkled liberally on food, don't ever ingest the essential cinnamon oil. Cinnamon spice can cause allergic reactions, but this isn't common.

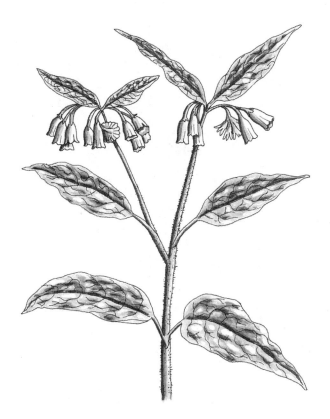

Comfrey (*Symphytum officinale*)

Lore: The early Greeks first used juicy comfrey root externally to treat wounds, believing that it encouraged torn flesh to grow back together.

Claims to fame: It's no accident that this herb's name sounds a lot like "comfort." In fact, comfrey is a great soother when it comes to minor wounds, burns, and other skin irritations. Scientists have discovered that the plant contains allantoin—a chemical that promotes the growth of new cells and thus speeds healing.

How to use: Mix 2 to 4 tablespoons of the powdered root with water to make a paste and apply it to the injured area. Change the comfrey preparation daily.

Cautions and recommendations: Comfrey is considered to be safe when applied externally. But don't ingest it. Though traditional herbalists once prescribed comfrey to relieve digestive problems, studies have shown that it may contain liver-damaging chemicals. As with any herbal remedy, discontinue use if your skin becomes red, itchy, or irritated after use.

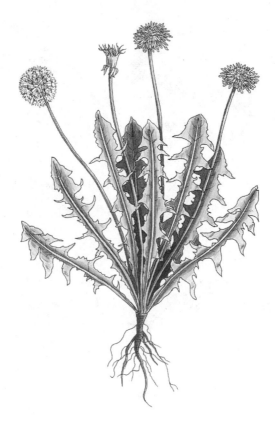

Dandelion (*Taraxacum officinale*)

Lore: During the Middle Ages, Europeans believed in the notion that the physical characteristics of plants revealed their healing value. Under this doctrine anything yellow—like dandelion—was linked to liver's yellow bile and considered a liver remedy.

Claims to fame: To a novice, it's just an annoying weed. To an herbalist, the entire dandelion—including the root—contains powerful medicines. Dandelion can boost appetite, soothe bellyaches, and reduce flatulence. It's also one of the safest diuretics that grows in the wild.

How to use: To make a tea, use 1 teaspoon of powdered root per cup of boiling water. Gently boil for 15 minutes. Cool. Drink up to 3 cups per day. For tinctures, follow package directions.

Cautions and recommendations: Do not take dandelion plant or root if you suffer from a bile duct obstruction. If you have gallstones, do not take dandelion until you have consulted with your health care practitioner. Also, repeated contact with dandelion may cause skin rashes in some people.

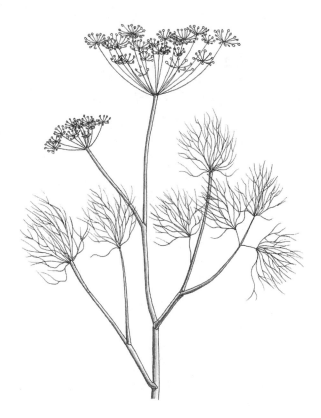

Dill (*Anethum graveolens*)

Lore: The ancient Greeks used this herb to quell hiccups. During the Middle Ages, dill was prized as protection against witchcraft.

Claims to fame: In a pickle when it comes to stomach troubles? Turn to dill. Centuries before refrigeration, herbalists discovered that adding dill to pickles increased their shelf life. Today, we know why: Dill inhibits the growth of food-spoiling microbes. That's also why dill can soothe some types of upset stomach. It's even gentle enough to soothe a colicky infant.

How to use: To make tea, steep 1 teaspoon of crushed dill seeds in a cup of boiling water for 10 minutes. Drink up to 3 cups a day. To ease colic, ask your baby's pediatrician about the proper dosage of weak dill tea.

Cautions and recommendations: Generally, dill's leaves, seeds, and seed oil are considered nontoxic. However, any type of food or beverage can cause an allergic reaction in some people. Though it's highly unlikely, some people develop a skin rash after eating or drinking preparations containing this herb.

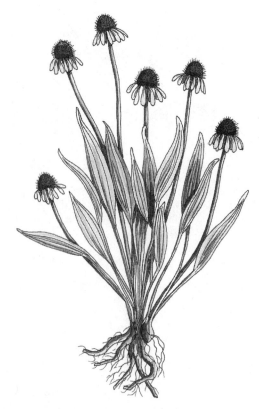

Echinacea (*Echinacea purpurea*)

Lore: Echinacea was the Plains Indians primary medicine. They applied root poultices to wounds, insect bites and stings, and snakebites.

Claims to fame: German research has shown that this daisylike plant powers up the immune system against viruses, bacteria, and fungi. That's why more and more doctors are suggesting that folks take this herb as a first treatment for colds and flu—before resorting to antibiotics. When applied as a poultice to wounds, sores, and burns, echinacea also may ward off infection and stimulate healing.

How to use: Herbalists advise taking this herb as a drink. Here's how: Add 1 teaspoon of tincture to 1 cup of water, juice, or tea. For a decoction (a gently simmered tea), add 1 teaspoon of root material per cup of boiling water and simmer for 15 minutes. Drink up to 3 cups of tea a day. Or buy premade tea bags and follow the package directions.

Cautions and recommendations: You get best results from echinacea if you take a week off after every two weeks of taking it. Avoid it altogether if you have multiple sclerosis, tuberculosis, AIDS, or HIV.

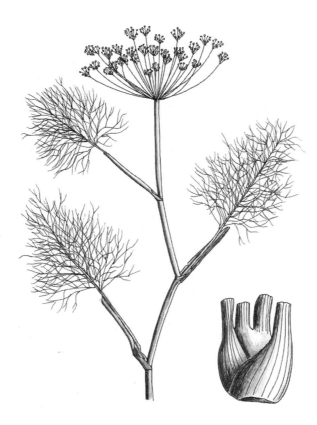

Fennel (*Foeniculum vulgare*)

Lore: Roman warriors took fennel to keep in good health.

Claims to fame: The seeds and the oil squeezed from them have been known to settle upset stomach and reduce flatulence. The herb might be able to reduce the stuffy nose that you get when you have a cold.

How to use: As a digestive aid, either chew ¼ to ½ teaspoon of seeds or make fennel tea. To make a pleasant licorice-flavored tea, use 1 to 2 teaspoons of crushed seeds per cup of boiling water. Steep for 10 minutes. Drink up to 3 cups a day.

Cautions and recommendations: Fennel can cause allergic reaction, though only rarely. If you are pregnant, doctors advise that you not take fennel.

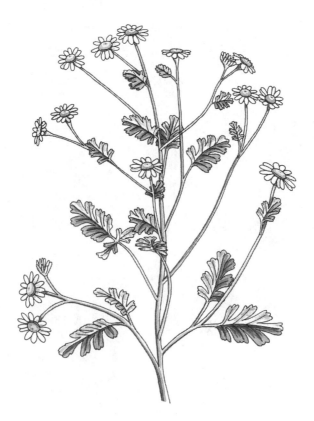

Feverfew (*Tanacetum parthenium*)

Lore: The word *feverfew* is actually a corruption of the Old English *featherfew*, a reference to the plant's feathery leaf borders.

Claims to fame: Since the 1980s, several studies have shown this herb to be effective at reducing the severity and frequency of migraines.

How to use: For migraine control, chew two fresh, frozen, or freeze-dried leaves a day or take a pill or capsule containing 85 milligrams of leaf material. Most people prefer pills, capsules, or tinctures to leaves since feverfew is quite bitter. Feverfew also can be used as an herbal tea, although it is also bitter.

Cautions and recommendations: Chewing feverfew leaves may cause irritation or ulcers around the lips, tongue, and mouth. Otherwise, this herb is considered safe for most adults but should not be taken by women who are pregnant or nursing or by adults 65 or older.

If you have high blood pressure, don't try to treat yourself and never discontinue taking a prescription medication. Before taking feverfew to reduce blood pressure, consult your physician.

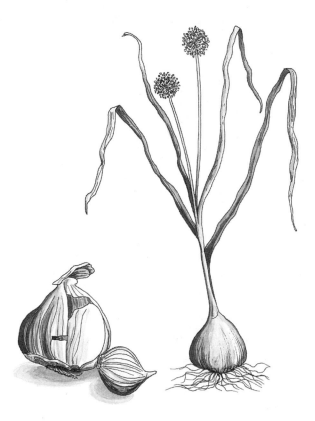

Garlic (*Allium sativum*)

Lore: Pyramid builders and Roman soldiers on long marches were fed a daily ration of garlic.

Claims to fame: Studies show that garlic helps protect against stomach cancer and reduces the risk of heart disease.

How to use: Fresh garlic should be crushed, chewed, or chopped. It may also be taken in pill form, as with the product Garlique. To fight illness or infection, chew a clove or two during the course of a day, or take the pills following the package directions. (Pills won't cause bad breath.)

Cautions and recommendations: In some people garlic can cause gastrointestinal upset if you eat more than four raw cloves a day. Garlic can also make a change in the beneficial bacteria of the bowel or lead to allergic reactions, and garlic odor can pervade the breath and the skin. The herb's anti-clotting action may prevent heart attacks and strokes, but medicinal amounts can cause problems for people with clotting disorders such as hemophilia or those who take anti-clotting drugs. If you have such conditions, ask your doctor before using garlic medicinally.

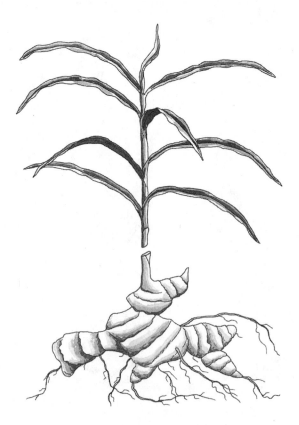

Ginger (*Zingiber officinale*)

Lore: Chinese emperor Shen Nung touted ginger as a cure for tetanus and leprosy.

Claims to fame: Research shows that ginger fights nausea better than Dramamine. And other studies show that it boosts the immune system's ability to fight infection. What's more, it helps prevent the blood clots that can trigger heart attacks and strokes. Ginger also can relieve headaches.

How to use: To relieve motion sickness, take 2 to 4 grams 30 minutes before departure. Capsules are usually the most convenient, but 12 ounces of ginger ale also provides some relief—that is, if it is made with real ginger. You can make ginger tea by mixing ½ teaspoon powdered root or 1 teaspoon grated root per cup of boiling water. Drink up to 3 cups a day.

Cautions and recommendations: Ginger is considered safe for most adults. It can help morning sickness, but pregnant or nursing women should not take ginger without the approval of their obstetricians. Also, some people develop heartburn or nausea after using large amounts of ginger. If this happens to you, try taking less or discontinue use.

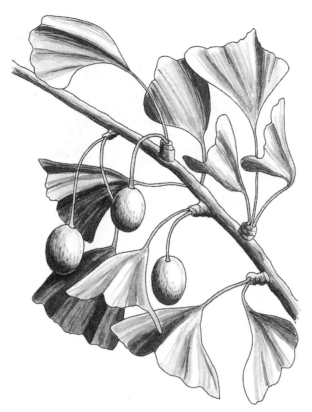

Ginkgo (*Ginkgo biloba*)

Lore: A relic of the dinosaur age, ginkgo is the oldest surviving tree on Earth.

Claims to fame: Ginkgo may increase blood flow to the brain, speeding recovery from stroke and improving memory. It also boosts blood flow to the heart (so it may prevent heart attack) as well as to the penis (which may relieve impotence in some men).

Studies also show that ginkgo can help treat chronic ringing in the ears (tinnitus), one form of hearing loss (cochlear deafness), and age-related vision loss (macular degeneration), as well as a condition called intermittent claudication. It may even help prevent asthma attacks and headaches.

How to use: Health food stores and pharmacies sell commercial preparations containing ginkgo extract. Follow package directions.

Cautions and recommendations: While it is harmless to take ginkgo to boost your brain power, don't try to self-treat any serious medical symptoms without consulting your physician. And never stop taking a prescription medication without your doctor's approval.

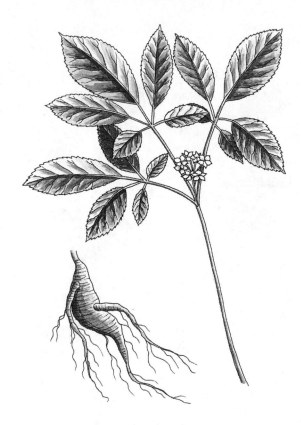

Ginseng (*Panax ginseng*)

Lore: One of Asia's most revered herbs, Confucius praised ginseng's healing powers more than 2,000 years ago.

Claims to fame: Until recently, Western scientists scoffed at ginseng claims. But evidence is mounting that the herb may help the body resist illness and damage caused by stress. Studies suggest that ginseng stimulates the immune system, helps reduce cholesterol levels, protects the liver from toxic substances, increases stamina, and improves nutrient absorption in the intestines.

How to use: Herb companies market ginseng teas, tablets, capsules, and tinctures. Follow package directions for dosage.

To make ginseng tea yourself, add ½ teaspoon of powdered root per cup of boiling water. Simmer for 10 minutes. Drink up to 2 cups per day.

Cautions and recommendations: Ginseng rarely causes side effects, but it's advisable to avoid caffeine while taking it. If you decide to use ginseng, start with a low dose. And as with most other herbs, ginseng shouldn't be taken by pregnant or nursing women without their doctors' approval.

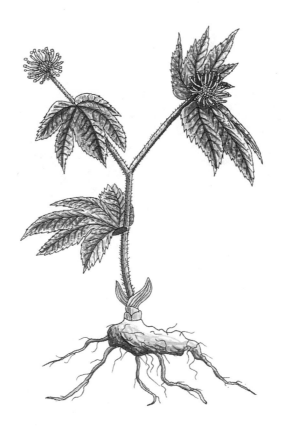

Goldenseal (*Hydrastis canadensis*)

Lore: A favorite Native American infection fighter, goldenseal was widely used to treat battle wounds during the Civil War.

Claims to fame: Herbalists consider goldenseal an effective remedy for soothing sore throats, easing the pain of canker sores, preventing the spread of various types of infection, and even curing diarrhea by killing the germs that cause it.

How to use: To make tea, use ½ to 1 teaspoon of powdered root per cup of boiling water and steep for 10 minutes. It has an unpleasant taste, but you can use it as a mouthwash or drink up to 2 cups a day. When using commercial preparations, such as tinctures or capsules, follow package directions. Never use more than the recommended amount.

Cautions and recommendations: Many herbalists recommend goldenseal, but further study needs to be done. Meanwhile, never take this herb if you are pregnant or have high blood pressure, heart disease, or glaucoma. It is best to take it for a limited time period—no more than a week or two—since as it accumulates in the body, it can become slightly toxic.

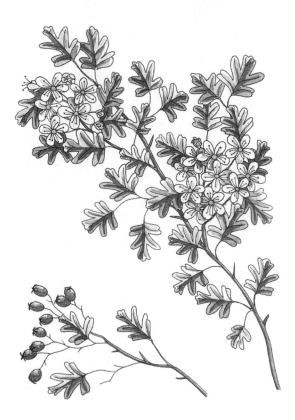

Hawthorn (*Crataegus* species)

Lore: The Romans placed hawthorn leaves in babies' cradles to ward off evil spirits.

Claims to fame: Hawthorn ranks as an impressive herb to help maintain your heart and boost blood flow. It works by dilating the blood vessels, especially those near the heart. Herbalists have used the bright red berries since the late nineteenth century. But scientists only recently discovered that the flowers contain important medicinal compounds. European doctors often prescribe hawthorn during initial stages of a heart problem.

How to use: To make a tea, mix 1 to 2 teaspoons of crushed leaves or fruits per cup of boiling water. Steep for 20 minutes. Drink up to 2 cups a day.

Cautions and recommendations: There are no known health risks. But Germany's Commission E says not to use the herb for more than six weeks at a time because it acts on the heart. And remember: Since a heart condition is serious, see a physician if you have swollen legs, heart pain, arm pain, or other symptoms of heart disorders.

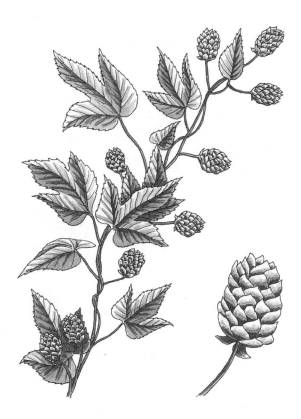

Hops (*Humulus lupulus*)

Lore: Until the sixteenth century, English brewers avoided using hops in their beers in the belief that the herb induced melancholy. That all ended when the extremely hoppy India Pale Ale was invented. The British controlled India and wanted to send beer to their troops. So they dumped a ton of hops into the brew to preserve the mixture for the long trip.

Claims to fame: Other than preserving beer and providing its bitter flavor and aroma, hops can help you get to sleep at night. Hops also have been known to treat moodiness, restlessness, and anxiety.

How to use: To make hop tea, use 1 to 2 teaspoons of the herb per cup of boiling water. Steep for 5 minutes. Hops taste pleasantly bitter. You can also make a sleeping pillow from hops by stuffing fabric with ¼ cup dried hops and then sewing up the opening. You can add other fragrant herbs as well. Lay your hops pillow underneath your regular pillow.

Cautions and recommendations: Hops are safe, and you can even take them with other herbal sedatives.

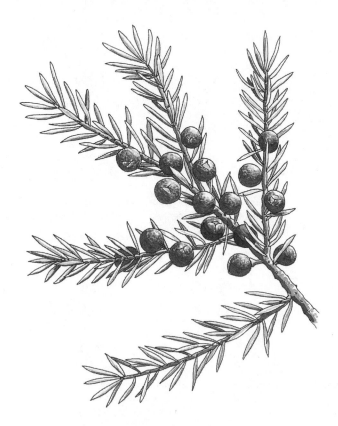

Juniper (*Juniperus communis*)

Lore: During the Middle Ages, Europeans believed that planting juniper beside the front door kept witches out.

Claims to fame: Juniper berries are sometimes helpful in easing upset stomach, indigestion, flatulence, and other stomach disorders. Juniper also may have anti-inflammatory properties, suggesting that it may have value in treating arthritis, and it has been used to treat bladder infection.

How to use: To make tea, mix 1 teaspoon of crushed berries per cup of boiling water. Steep for 10 to 20 minutes. Though you can drink up to 2 cups per day (for no more than six weeks), the tea is very strong. You can use a tincture or capsules instead.

Cautions and recommendations: Like coffee, juniper can make you urinate frequently and has been known to cause kidney irritation. So avoid juniper if you are pregnant or have kidney disease.

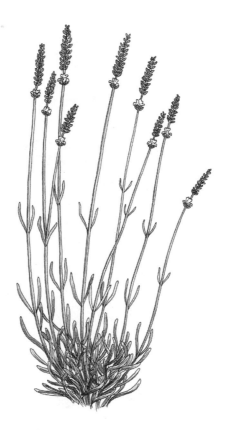

Lavender (*Lavandula angustifolia*)

Lore: Lavender was used to perfume the baths of the Romans. It has been used as a folk remedy for at least 1,000 years.

Claims to fame: The sedative powers of lavender flowers can soothe mood disturbances, such as nervous stomach, flatulence, restlessness, and insomnia—and it's known as a germ fighter.

How to use: Put lavender in a cloth bag in your bath, using about a handful, or add 2 to 4 drops of essential oil to your bathwater.

Cautions and recommendations: Lavender can be taken in conjunction with other sedatives or anti-flatulent herbs.

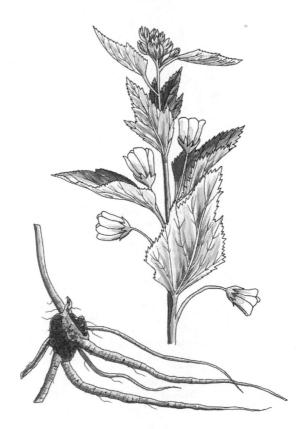

Marsh Mallow (*Althaea officinalis*)

Lore: Marsh mallow root is mentioned in the Old Testament, so its reputation as a healing herb has a long history.

Claims to fame: The root can alleviate sore throat, dry cough, and mild stomach inflammation. When applied to the skin, marsh mallow gel may help soothe skin irritation or rashes.

How to use: You can make a sweet tea by boiling ½ to 1 teaspoon of chopped or crushed root per cup of water for 10 to 15 minutes. Drink up to 3 cups a day.

To prepare marsh mallow for external use, powder the root very fine and add enough water to make a gooey gel. Apply the gel directly to superficial wounds or sunburn. If you have a serious wound or burn, consult your doctor.

Cautions and recommendations: Some experts believe that marsh mallow root can slow the absorption of other medications. If marsh mallow causes minor discomfort, use less or stop using it altogether.

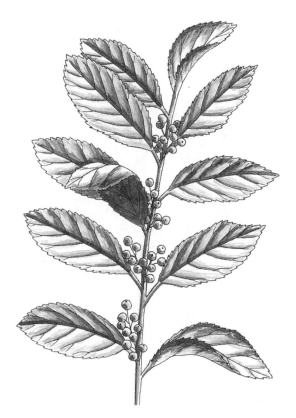

Maté (*Ilex paraguariensis*)

Lore: More than 300 years ago, Jesuit priests noticed that South American Indians appeared immune to scurvy. The priests decided that the Indians must be protected by the tea that they drank out of cups made from calabash gourds. They named it *maté*, from the Spanish word for gourd.

Claims to fame: Think of it as a strong cup of coffee. Just like the coffee bean, the maté plant contains the stimulant caffeine. People take the herb to perk up mentally and physically.

How to use: To make a strong, bitter tea, mix 1 teaspoon of dried herb per cup of boiling water. Steep for 10 minutes. Drink up to 3 cups a day. To mask the bitter taste, add lemon and honey.

Cautions and recommendations: Maté should not be given to children under age 2. For older children and people over 65, start with low-strength preparations and increase strength, if necessary.

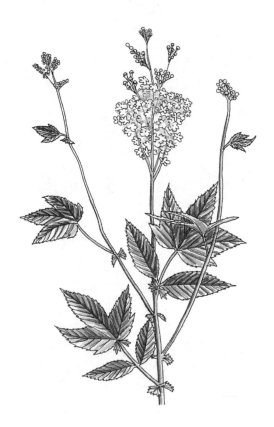

Meadowsweet (*Filipendula ulmaria*)

Lore: Meadowsweet was one of the Druids' sacred herbs.

Claims to fame: Even the name of this herb connotes calm. And that's exactly what it does for the stomach—helps reduce nausea. The herb contains salicin, which gets converted in the stomach into the main ingredient in aspirin, salicylic acid. Like aspirin, this herb can cool a fever and numb pain. But unlike aspirin, this natural painkiller is much less irritating to the stomach than its purer cousin.

How to use: To make a tea, mix a cup of boiling water with 1 to 2 teaspoons of dried meadowsweet. Let it steep for 10 to 15 minutes and drink three times a day. If you buy the herb in tincture form, swallow 25 to 50 drops three times a day.

Cautions and recommendations: Do not give meadowsweet to children under 18. Like aspirin, meadowsweet contains salicin that has been associated with Reye's syndrome, a rare but potentially fatal illness that affects the brain and liver.

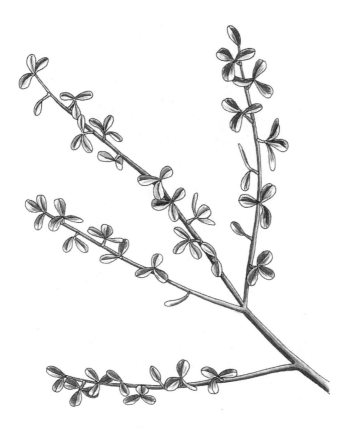

Myrrh (*Commiphora* species)

Lore: First used by the ancient Egyptians in embalming mixtures, myrrh became the all-purpose Biblical aromatic for perfumes, funerals, and insect repellents. Perhaps the herb is best known from the nativity story when the three Wise Men presented the incense as a gift to the baby Jesus.

Claims to fame: While people back in Biblical times used the perfumelike myrrh on a corpse as part of burial preparations, today, myrrh is used as a topical treatment for skin infections, mouth inflammations, tooth decay, and gum disease.

How to use: For a mouthwash, steep 1 teaspoon of powdered herb and 1 teaspoon of boric acid or salt in 1 pint of boiling water. Let stand for 30 minutes then strain. Wait for it to cool before gargling.

Cautions and recommendations: Avoid ingestion, as some herbalists think that large amounts of myrrh may cause laxative action.

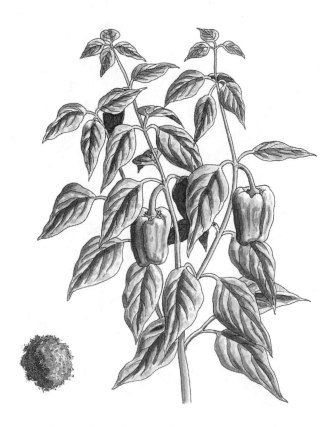

Paprika (*Capsicum* species)

Lore: Paprika and other varieties of peppers have probably been cultivated for hundreds of years in places such as Africa, India, and the tropical Americas, where they were used to soothe head colds and stomachaches.

Claims to fame: Paprika, a pepper from the cayenne family, contains small amounts of the healing oil capsaicin. When applied to the skin, a paprika solution can ease nerve pain. Cayenne is hot to more than your tongue. It can also keep your skin warm, preventing frostbite.

How to use: Use commercial products containing capsaicin (the active ingredient in paprika) as directed. To keep your hands and feet warm in the cold winter outdoors, sprinkle some in your socks and gloves—but be aware that it can stain clothing.

Cautions and recommendations: If you are allergic to cayenne or paprika, don't use it. Also, remember that pepper oil can burn your eyes, nose, and mouth. Wash it off your hands after applying it to other areas of your body. Overexposure can produce pain, dizziness, and rapid pulse even when used externally.

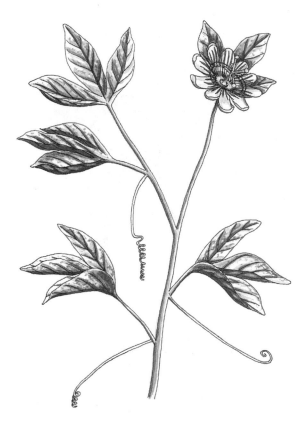

Passionflower (*Passiflora incarnata*)

Lore: The Incas brewed a tonic tea from passionflower.

Claims to fame: Passionflower can soothe nerves and restlessness.

How to use: To make a pleasant-tasting tea that can help you relax or fall asleep, use 1 teaspoon of dried leaves per cup of boiling water. Steep for 10 to 15 minutes. For insomnia, drink a cup before bed. For other uses, drink up to 3 cups a day.

Cautions and recommendations: The medical literature contains no reports of harm from passionflower. However, the flower does contain one or more harmala compounds, which are uterine stimulants. Whole passionflower has not been associated with miscarriage, but it is prudent for pregnant women to stay away from the herb. Use only this species medicinally. The closely related blue passionflower can be toxic.

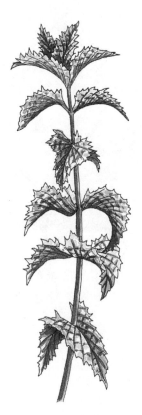

Peppermint (*Mentha piperita*)

Lore: Mint was mentioned as a stomach soother in the *Ebers Papyrus*, the world's oldest surviving medical text.

Claims to fame: There are more perks to an after-dinner mint than just fresh breath. In fact, the herb that flavors these popular candies has long been revered as a stomach soother. What's more, this herb contains menthol, which relieves sinus and chest congestion. Peppermint leaves also are taken to relieve flatulence and spasms of the gastrointestinal tract and bile ducts. Peppermint oil is used as a treatment for irritable colon.

How to use: For tea, steep 1 teaspoon of fresh mint leaves or 1 to 2 teaspoons of dried leaves per cup of boiling water for 10 minutes. Drink up to 4 cups per day. For wounds, try an herbal bath. Fill a cloth bag with a few handfuls of dried or fresh herb and let the water run over it.

Cautions and recommendations: Peppermint in tea or candy is generally considered safe for adults, but don't give it to infants or very young children. Both peppermint essential oil and pure menthol are poisonous, and neither should be taken internally.

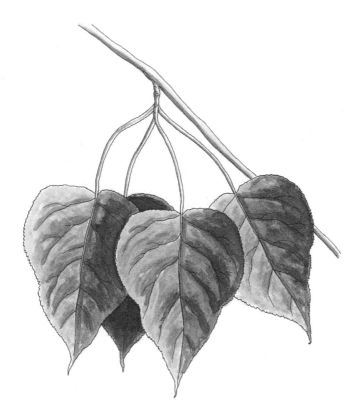

Poplar (*Populus* species)

Lore The Greeks thought that this tree came from the Heliades, the grief-stricken sisters of Phaëthon, who saw their brother fall from the sky as he drove the sun's chariot. The sisters were turned into poplar trees, and their tears fell in a stream that became amber.

Claims to fame: Money doesn't grow on trees, but antibiotics do. The tiny buds from the poplar tree have a natural antibacterial agent that can help heal and disinfect cuts, hemorrhoids, frostbite, and sunburn.

How to use: Poplar buds can be made into a cream or a salve.

Cautions and recommendations: If you are allergic to poplar buds, propolis, Peruvian balsam, or aspirin, avoid this herb.

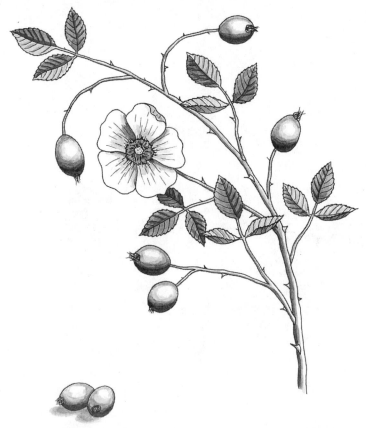

Rose (*Rosa gallica, R. centifolia*)

Lore: Roses were a favorite of the ancient Egyptians, who used the fragrant petals as air fresheners and the rose water as perfume.

Claims to fame: When drunk in a tea, rose hips (the ripened fruit) can soothe a sore throat.

How to use: You can make a tea by mixing 2 to 3 teaspoons of dried, chopped rose hips per cup of boiling water. Steep for 10 minutes. Drink as needed.

Cautions and recommendations: Some people believe that rose hips can treat more symptoms, especially vitamin C deficiencies.

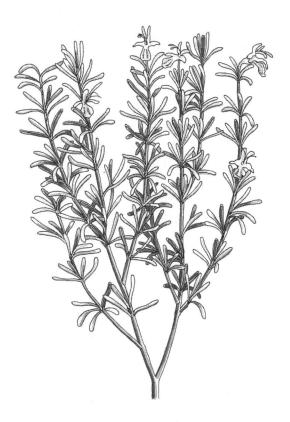

Rosemary (*Rosmarinus officinalis*)

Lore: During the plague of 1665, rosemary was carried in the handles of walking sticks and pouches to be sniffed when traveling through afflicted areas.

Claims to fame: Long before refrigeration, the ancients noticed that wrapping meat in crushed rosemary leaves not only flavored it nicely but also preserved it. Meats spoil partly because of a process called oxidation, which turns their fats rancid. Rosemary oil retards spoilage and compares favorably with commercial preservatives. Rosemary also relaxes smooth muscles like those of the digestive tract and uterus, which may make it effective at relieving indigestion and menstrual cramps.

How to use: Make a tea by steeping 1 teaspoon of crushed leaves in a cup of boiling water for 10 to 15 minutes. Drink up to 3 cups a day.

Cautions and recommendations: In the amounts used for cooking or in teas, rosemary is safe. But never drink rosemary essential oil—it's toxic. Opt for the dried or fresh herb instead. If you're pregnant, you should avoid using the herb medicinally, although you can use it as a seasoning.

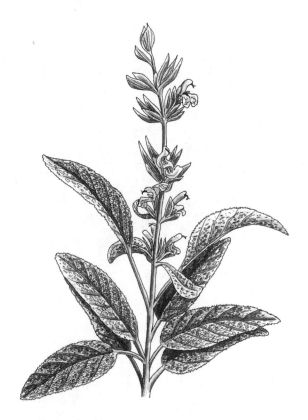

Sage (*Salvia officinalis*)

Lore: Ancient physicians ascribed marvelous healing and preventive powers to sage. There was a Latin saying in the Middle Ages that translates, "Why should a man die when sage grows in his garden?"

Claims to fame: This is natural germ warfare. Sage leaf as well as the juice from it has natural antibacterial and antifungal agents. It can be used as an astringent for sore throat and germs.

How to use: To make a tea, pour 1 cup of boiling water over 1 teaspoon of dried leaves. Steep for 10 minutes. Drink up to 3 cups per day. Or, add honey for sore throat and gargle the mixture. Sage tastes warm, aromatic, and somewhat pungent.

Cautions and recommendations: Sage essential oil contains relatively high levels of one toxic chemical called thujone. In large amounts thujone causes a variety of symptoms culminating in convulsions. But the herb is safe when used as a spice. Sage essential oil may cause toxicity and should not be ingested. Commission E recommends that pregnant women not ingest sage or its extracts.

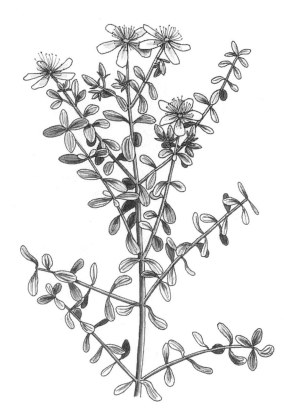

St.-John's-wort (*Hypericum perforatum*)

Lore: The herb begins blooming around the birthday of St. John, which is June 24. *Wort* is a Middle English word for herb.

Claims to fame: Experts say this herb reduces inflammation when swallowed, but it's more often used to treat anxiety, tension, irritability, and depression. The herb also may ease fibrositis (inflammation of fibrous muscles, which causes pain and stiffness mainly in the muscles used for movement) or sciatica (inflammation or injury to the sciatic nerve, which causes pain that travels from the back or thigh through the leg and into the foot and toes). You can also apply it to the skin to reduce swelling, relieve varicose veins, and heal bruises and mild burns, including sunburn.

How to use: To make a tea, mix a cup of boiling water with 1 to 2 teaspoons of St.-John's-wort and steep for 10 to 15 minutes. Drink this tea three times a day. If you buy the herb in tincture form, follow recommendations on the package since strengths will vary.

Cautions and recommendations: Experts suspect that St.-John's-wort may cause sun sensitivity.

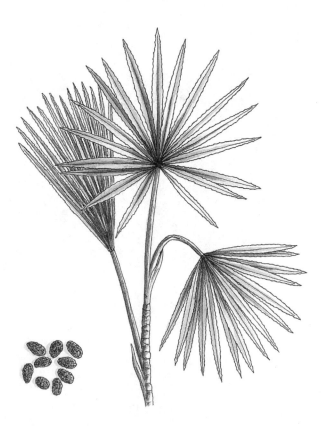

Saw Palmetto (*Serenoa repens*)

Lore: Saw palmetto's healing properties were discovered strictly by accident. Early settlers on the southeastern coast of the United States noticed that animals that ate the berries were healthier than animals that did not. So the settlers decided to give the berries a try themselves.

Claims to fame: The saw palmetto berry helps the urination problems associated with enlarged prostate due to benign causes, such as benign prostatic hyperplasia, or BPH, which affects men over the age of 50.

How to use: For relief of symptoms related to prostate problems, the recommended dose is 160 milligrams twice a day. It's impossible to obtain that dose from plant material; it would require eating ½ pound of berries a day. But you can take saw palmetto capsules that provide a high enough dose.

Cautions and recommendations: Never try to self-medicate a prostate problem. Alert your doctor if you're having prostate or urinary tract problems. And don't begin taking this herb without your physician's permission. In rare cases, saw palmetto can cause stomach problems.

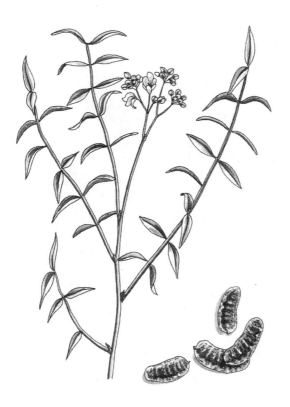

Senna (*Cassia senna*)

Lore: During the ninth century, the great caliph of Baghdad became dissatisfied with the medicines available in his court, particularly the laxatives that caused him severe abdominal distress. So his physician brought a host of new medicines to the court, including the laxative senna.

Claims to fame: These dried leaves and pods are a powerful laxative.

How to use: Because of senna's disgusting taste, herbalists generally discourage using the plant material and instead recommend over-the-counter products containing it. Follow package directions.

Cautions and recommendations: Avoid this herb if you have a heart arrhythmia. Also, don't double it up with laxatives, diuretics, or steroids.

This is a powerful laxative that should only be used as a last resort to relieve constipation, and it's advisable to take an anti-flatulence herb, such as fennel, mint, or coriander with it. Most commercial preparations include the anti-flatulence herb as well. Reduce the dosage if you get cramps. Don't use it if you have Crohn's disease, colitis, or abdominal pain.

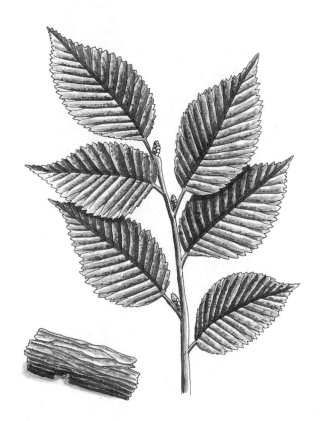

Slippery Elm (*Ulmus rubra*)

Lore: Native Americans taught early European settlers how to use slippery elm, and it quickly became one of the most important home remedies in colonial America.

Claims to fame: Perhaps the ultimate soother, Native Americans used slippery elm both as a food and as a treatment for wounds, sore throats, coughing, upset stomachs, and infant colic. Later, slippery elm sore throat lozenges became a fixture in home medicine chests.

How to use: To make a poultice for minor wounds, first cleanse the affected area. Then stir enough water into powdered bark to make a paste and apply to the wound. Change the poultice daily.

To take slippery elm internally, make a tea. Use 1 to 3 teaspoons of powdered bark per cup of water. (Blend a little water in first to prevent lumpiness.) Bring to a boil and simmer for 15 minutes. Drink up to 3 cups a day.

Cautions and recommendations: As with any herbal remedy, discontinue use if you develop allergic reactions such as skin rashes or itching.

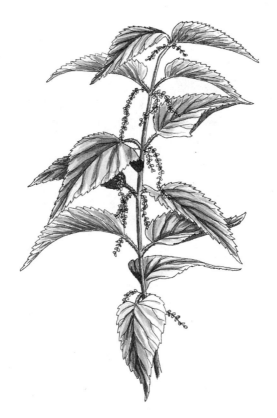

Stinging Nettle (*Urtica urens* and *U. dioica*)

Lore: Roman soldiers flailed themselves with nettles in cold climates because the herb's sting warmed their skin.

Claims to fame: Painful though it is, this herb can reduce joint swelling if you're willing to flail it against your skin. It can also be made into a tea or juice to help treat the pain of gout and possibly help with prostate enlargement.

How to use: For juice, process fresh root in a blender or juicer. To make a tea, use 1 to 2 teaspoons of dried herbs per cup of boiling water. Steep for 10 minutes. Drink up to 2 cups a day for urinary tract infections.

Cautions and recommendations: This herb's sting is its major problem. If you harvest it, wear gloves, a long-sleeved shirt, and long pants.

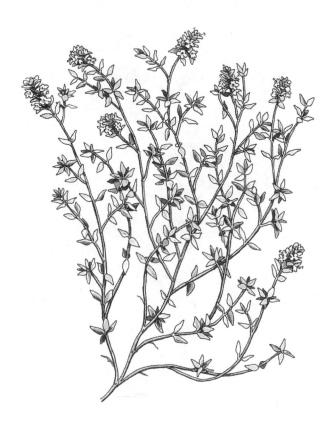

Thyme (*Thymus zygis* and *T. vulgaris*)

Lore: According to ancient tradition, if a girl wears a corsage of wild thyme flowers, it means that she is looking for a sweetheart.

Claims to fame: Because it can kill bacteria and soothe bronchial spasms, thyme is used to treat bronchitis and other upper respiratory inflammations.

How to use: For minor cuts and scrapes, make a poultice of fresh leaves and press the wound as soon as possible. Once the wound has been thoroughly washed and cleaned, apply a few drops of thyme tincture as an antiseptic before bandaging it.

To make a tea to help settle the stomach or soothe a cough, use 1 teaspoon of dried herb per cup of boiling water. Steep for 10 minutes. Drink up to 3 cups a day. Syrup with thyme is good for coughs and is available at many health food stores. Be sure to follow package directions.

Cautions and recommendations: Although thyme is available as an essential oil, do not take it internally. Instead, always opt for the fresh or dried herb.

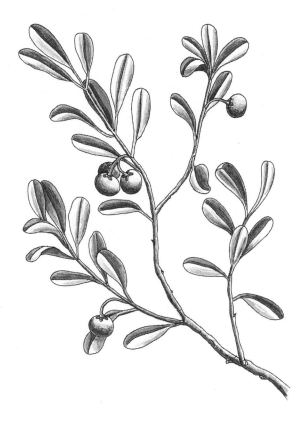

Uva Ursi (*Arctostaphylos uva ursi*)

Lore: This herb was largely ignored by Western herbalists until Marco Polo reported that Chinese physicians were using it as a diuretic.

Claims to fame: This ground-cover herb is used to treat bladder infections. It is believed to contain a powerful antiseptic that activates when in the urinary tract. Once there, it kills bacteria, removes infectious material, reduces inflammation, and may even strengthen the urinary tract lining.

How to use: To minimize the unpleasant taste of this highly astringent herb, soak the leaves in cold water overnight. Toss out that batch of water. Then, to make a strong tea to help treat urinary symptoms or diarrhea, simmer 1 teaspoon of the herb leaves in a cup of boiling water for 10 minutes. Drink up to 3 cups per day.

Cautions and recommendations: Uva ursi can sometimes cause nausea and vomiting in children and in adults with sensitive stomachs. Check with your doctor first if you are on some other medication that might make your urine acidic. Don't use this herb for more than one week, because after that, it can irritate your kidneys.

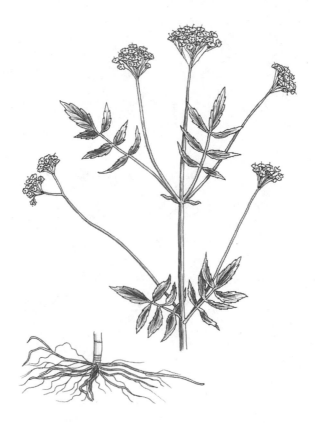

Valerian (*Valeriana officinalis*)

Lore: In the original story of the Pied Piper of Hamelin, the flute player was thought to have used music and valerian root, an herb with hypnotic chemicals similar to catnip, to lure away the town's children.

Claims to fame: Studies show that valerian has tranquilizing and sedative properties similar to those of Valium. The added benefit is that valerian is nonaddictive. And it doesn't have the side effects of dizziness, blurred vision, drowsiness, or poor physical performance the next day that prescription sleeping pills can have.

How to use: To make valerian tea, use 2 teaspoons of chopped root per cup of boiling water. Steep for 10 to 15 minutes. Add lemon and sugar or honey or mix with a beverage. Drink 1 cup before bed. If using a tincture, take ½ to 1 teaspoon before bed.

Cautions and recommendations: Don't give valerian to children under age 2. For older children and people over 65, start with low-strength preparations and increase strength if necessary. Consult your physician for help with ongoing sleep problems.

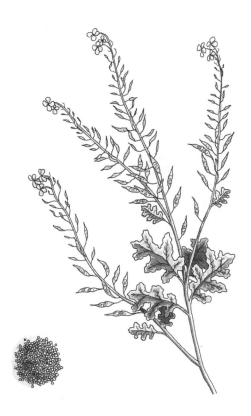

White Mustard (*Sinapis alba*)

Lore: The English name *mustard* comes from the Latin *mustum ardens*, or "burning must," which refers to the early French practice of grinding the pungent seeds with grape must (the still-fermenting juice of wine grapes).

Claims to fame: White mustard seed is usually made into a paste and plastered onto an inflamed joint or sore muscle.

How to use: To make the paste, mix 4 tablespoons of powdered mustard seed with warm water and 4 tablespoons of flour (to lessen the heat). Apply for 5 to 10 minutes to children and 10 to 15 minutes to adults, but remove after that, as it may burn the skin.

Cautions and recommendations: Long-term use can cause skin irritation. Also, avoid using on children younger than age six or on people with kidney problems.

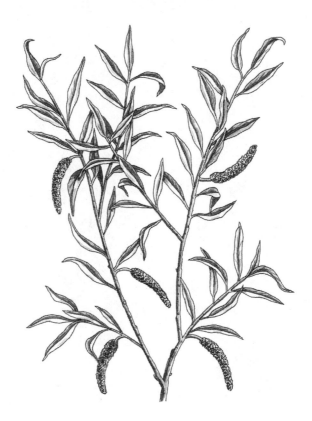

White Willow (*Salix alba*)

Lore: Chinese physicians have used white willow bark to relieve pain since 500 B.C.

Claims to fame: The tree's inner bark contains natural aspirin-like substances. It's used to relieve pain, cool fevers, and soothe headaches.

How to use: For a pain-, fever-, and inflammation-relieving infusion, soak 1 teaspoon of powdered bark per cup of cold water for 8 hours. Strain. Drink up to 3 cups a day. White willow tastes bitter and astringent. Add honey and lemon or mix it with an herbal tea.

Cautions and recommendations: Scientists have yet to nail down this herb's side effects, but it could cause stomach upset as aspirin does.

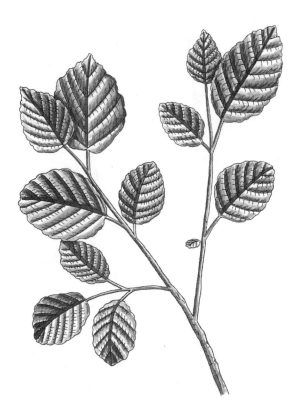

Witch Hazel (*Hamamelis virginiana*)

Lore: Native Americans used the limbs of this plant to make bows. In the 1840s, an Oneida medicine man introduced this herb's medicinal uses to a patent-medicine entrepreneur. It has been a mainstay of medicine cabinets ever since.

Claims to fame: Many Native American tribes made a tea of witch hazel and used it as a treatment for colds, fevers, and sore throats and as a liniment for relief from menstrual cramps. They also rubbed the tea on cuts, bruises, insect stings, and sore muscles and joints. Even some mainstream doctors who are skeptical of herbs recommend this traditional treatment for cuts, bruises, hemorrhoids, and rashes. More than a million gallons of witch hazel is sold in the United States annually.

How to use: Commercial witch hazel water should only be used externally because it is made with rubbing alcohol. Moisten a clean cloth and apply it to minor cuts, bruises, and other minor skin irritations.

Cautions and recommendations: As with all herbs, discontinue use if any sensitivity develops.

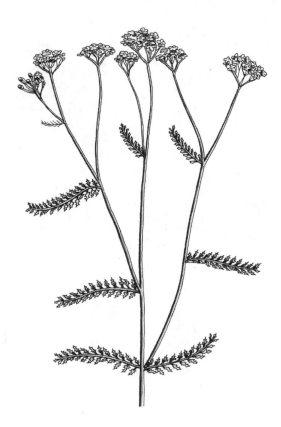

Yarrow (*Achillea millefolium*)

Lore: Long before settlers came to America, Europeans used yarrow to cast spells and make love charms.

Claims to fame: This herb helps sinus congestion, fever, colds, and flu. Women can drink yarrow tea to relieve menstrual cramps.

How to use: To make a tea that aids circulation and pain relief, use 1 teaspoon of dried herb per cup of boiling water. Steep for 10 to 15 minutes. Drink up to 3 cups per day. You can also apply the tea externally to cleanse wounds and inflammations.

Cautions and recommendations: People who are allergic to ragweed might develop a rash, sneezing, headache, or nausea if they use yarrow.

part 3

Nature's Best Healers

Quick Access

to Pill-Free Remedies

Aches and Pains

There should be a mirror up there on the painkiller shelves because you may already be holding the real key to pain relief—in your mind.

For years doctors have been prescribing painkilling drugs to people afflicted with chronic backaches, headaches, and joint aches. And much of the time, the medications worked. Backs unkinked, heads cleared, and joint pain backed off. But stomachs have not been so grateful; erosion of the stomach lining is an all-too-common side effect of painkiller therapy.

So it's big news to think that there's a way to chase chronic pain without drugs. It's even bigger news to know that nature's best pain reliever may be your own mind—if you know how to use it.

A prestigious panel of experts organized by the National Institutes of Health in Bethesda, Maryland, has declared that deep relaxation may help relieve chronic pain as readily as drugs and surgery. This marks a major departure from traditional medical thought in the United States. For the first time ever, some of the most renowned medical experts in America officially recognize that relaxation is a valid treatment—perhaps even the treatment to try first—for lower-back pain, headaches, arthritis, and other chronically painful disorders. And, unlike painkillers and operations, this kind of relaxation requires fewer doctor visits and has fewer side effects. Nobody has ever suffered an eroded stomach lining as a result of sitting down and focusing on his breathing.

Lest you think that this declaration comes from some companies trying to sell cassettes of recorded water sounds, understand that relaxation as pain treatment was embraced by truly mainstream doctors reporting in the renowned *Journal of the American Medical Association*.

Just what type of relaxation are we talking about? It's not the kind of relaxation that you get from vegging out in front of reruns of *Sisters* with a cup of tea. It goes deeper than that. In fact, people who meditate might recognize some of the relaxation techniques discussed here. But you don't have to attain Nirvana to get relief. The total relaxation that we're talking about falls somewhere between the couch and the meditation pillow.

Troubleshooting Guide
for the Reluctant Relaxer

Relaxing isn't easy at first, and some folks may be uncomfortable with the idea of deep relaxation or meditation. So here's a beginner's guide to total relaxation.

You won't have to twist yourself into a pretzel, subscribe to a new spiritual theory, or do anything far out. This is about relaxation, and it feels good. Promise.

Problem: I just can't seem to relax on command.

Solution: Sure you can. It just takes practice. "Relaxation is an acquired skill," says Dennis C. Turk, Ph.D., professor of anesthesiology and pain research at the University of Washington School of Medicine in Seattle. He suggests imagining that your muscles are melting like butter. Or, try thinking about warm water flowing over your body. You also might create a comforting scene in your mind, switching each day to a new locale until you find one that works. "There might be a beach scene, a snow scene, or a scene of sitting pleasantly in a fine restaurant listening to the tinkling of glasses and conversation," says Dr. Turk.

Problem: I have trouble with visualization. Me lying on a beach? I can't imagine that.

Solution: Put a visualization tape in your stereo. "Find the tape that works for you," says Dr. Turk. "What's relaxing and pleasant for me may not be for you. For example, once I made a tape for a guy to help him envision skiing down a mountain on a lovely, cold, sunny day. It was right for him, but to me, a cold, sunny day is when I'd like to be inside by a fireplace."

If store-bought audiotapes don't do the trick, make your own relaxing tape, using your voice or a friend's. Involve all your senses in creating an image, Dr. Turk says.

"Try to make it as engaging and involving as possible. For example, talk about the sounds of birds, the smell of flowers, and the feel of the breeze against your skin," says Dr. Turk. "Add a drink of lemonade next to you so you'll taste the tart lemon. Try to make it as vivid as possible because the more distracting it is, the more engaging it is, and the better the effect it's going to have."

Problem: I just get frustrated with relaxation audiotapes. They're too new-agey for my taste.

Solution: Another trick that works well is to focus on a scent, a picture, or a candle flame.

Or sweat away your physical tension with exercise, suggests Margaret A. Caudill, M.D., Ph.D., co-director of the Arnold Pain Center at Beth Israel Deaconess Medical Center in Boston and author of *Managing Pain before It Manages You.* Downshifting through yoga, tai chi, or gentle stretches also helps.

Stress reduction expert Jon Kabat-Zinn, Ph.D., director of the University of Massachusetts Medical Center's Stress Reduction Clinic in Worcester and author of *Full Catastrophe Living,* recommends a body scan. "Bring moment-to-moment awareness to each region of your body, starting with your feet, then moving up your legs and torso, then to your hands and arms, and ending with your neck and head," he suggests. "As you encounter areas of discomfort and pain, try intentionally relaxing and softening around them. Try to sense your breath moving in and out through all regions of your body." Whatever method you choose, you should not expect instant results. Cultivating relaxation takes a certain amount of effort and discipline, especially in the early stages of learning.

Problem: I'm in too much pain to think of a pretty scene.

Solution: Try something easier, suggests Dr. Turk, like focusing on your breathing as you think of the letters c-a-l-m in blue neon light. "That's what works for me," he says.

You also may want to change positions—perhaps try sitting instead of lying down, or vice versa, Dr. Caudill says.

If you can't disregard your pain, you might try the Lamaze approach—breathe into it. "Actively breathe deeply into the area of pain and then feel as if the pain is rushing out with each exhalation," says Jim Spira, Ph.D., a licensed psychologist and director of the Institute for Health Psychology in San Diego.

Problem: Errant thoughts keep diverting my attention.

Solution: If your mind still chatters like a teenager on the phone, keep a notepad nearby so that you can jot down your thoughts. Eventually, you'll run out of ideas and worries, and your mind will clear. Or try visualizing a basket and imagining that you are stuffing all your concerns and pain into it—and closing the lid, Dr. Caudill says. Whatever you do, don't blame yourself if you can't clear your mind, she adds. "If you judge yourself, you create a feeling of failure. And you don't need that."

Problem: I feel vulnerable when I lie there with my eyes closed.

Solution: Keep your eyes open, leave the lights on, and lock the door. Remember, this isn't as difficult as it may seem. Do what makes you feel relaxed and comfortable.

Learn to Ignore the Buzz

It's a simple state of mind to achieve—if you know the tricks. First, you break the train of everyday thoughts that induce stress by focusing on the repetition of a word, sound, thought, or breath. Second, you passively disregard other thoughts. Think of them as bumblebees buzzing around your head on a summer day. If you swat at them, you'll only make the bees angry and persistent. But if you ignore them, they'll buzz a bit and move on.

Like stress, relaxation works from the inside out. As you unwind, your body makes a 180-degree turn, switching from arousal to recuperation. Muscles relax, breathing slows, and your metabolism and blood pressure drop, says Herbert Benson, M.D., president of the Mind/Body Institute and director of behavioral medicine at Beth Israel Deaconess Medical Center/Harvard Medical School in Boston.

In contrast, when we're anxious, our bodies prepare to fight or flee. Muscles tense, blood pressures rise, breathing races, and our pain thresholds fall. It doesn't take too many traffic jams and toddler tantrums for our bodies to be tighter than our clothes after the holidays.

Deep relaxation can short-circuit not only pain but also the emotions that accompany pain, says Dennis C. Turk, Ph.D., professor of anesthesiology and pain research at the University of Washington School of Medicine in Seattle. "The worst thing is to feel helpless—that there's nothing you can do—like when you wake up at 3:00 A.M. with a terrible headache or back pain. You lie in bed thinking about how miserable you are. If you can use these types of relaxation techniques to gain some sense of control, that in itself can reduce some of the stress and discomfort you experience," he says.

Relaxed: How to Get There from Here

"Oh, just relax!" That sounds easy, but for many of us it's not. To succeed, start by lying down or sitting (with your back fairly straight, feet flat on the floor, and hands in your lap) in a darkened room, preferably one that's quiet and without distractions.

Close your eyes and breathe through your nose. Concentrate on your breathing. Make sure that you are "belly-breathing"—that is, forcing your belly to expand before your chest rises. This ensures that you are

*Herbal*SOLUTION

Tonic Soothes Muscle Soreness

For massaging out muscle tension, Mary Bove, a naturopathic physician, licensed midwife, and director of the Brattleboro Naturopathic Clinic in Vermont, recommends this herbal massage oil. Start with 1 cup of extra-virgin olive oil or almond oil (available in most health food stores). Pour the oil into a bottle or jar and add the following herbs in tincture form: 1 ounce of cramp bark, ½ ounce of lobelia, and ¼ ounce of willow bark or wintergreen. (If you don't have wintergreen tincture, Dr. Bove says to substitute 30 drops of wintergreen oil.) These ingredients are available at most health food stores and through mail order.

bringing air deep into your lungs. As you breathe out, imagine all tension in your body and mind leaving through your breath.

At this point—just like at night when your head hits the pillow— you'll probably notice your mind darting from every unpaid bill to every gained pound to every unfinished task.

That's where the repetition of a word such as "one," "peace," "love," or "shalom" comes in, says Dr. Benson.

You can focus on the rhythm of your breath, riding its waves as if you were a raft bobbing on a river. When extraneous thoughts show up, reel them in like fish. Catch them, admire them, then plop them on the bottom of the boat and return to fishing, er, relaxing.

You might find it easier to unwind if you simply reflect on what you are thinking and feeling right now, in the present moment. Audiotapes that help you cultivate this awareness (sometimes by painting a serene scene, such as a mountain, a lake, or a stand of trees) can help beginners, says Jon Kabat-Zinn, Ph.D., director of the University of Massachusetts Medical Center's Stress Reduction Clinic in Worcester and author of *Full Catastrophe Living.* "Guided meditation tapes are like training wheels; once you learn, you don't need them," he says. "Even so, many

(continued on page 122)

Hedge against Garden Aches

Baby green shoots and brown loamy earth feed the soul, but too much troweling and digging can make the rest of you feel awful.

"Just about all movement in a garden involves bending forward, which makes back muscles overstretch," says Judith Lasater, Ph.D., physical therapist and author of *Relax and Renew: Restful Yoga for Stressful Times*.

To relieve the strain on your spine, experts suggest a mild back bend that not only helps open up the front of your spine but also releases tension from back muscles by letting the full weight of your back and body rest supported on the floor. It also allows the front of your chest and rib cage to expand, allowing deeper, fuller breathing.

Take your time folding a regular-size bath towel properly, since this affects whether you end up feeling comfortable. Start by folding it in half lengthwise to form a long, skinny rectangle. Next, fold one of the skinny ends over about 6 inches, then roll it firmly until the whole towel is rolled. If your back is particularly stiff, only roll it halfway. Set it on the floor.

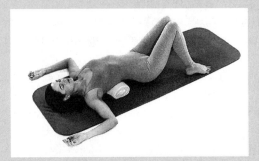

Lie on your back with the rolled towel positioned crosswise under your spine and just below your shoulder blades. Bend your knees with your feet flat on the floor, and rest your arms at your sides. You should be very comfortable and find relaxing very easy. (If you feel tension or pain in your back, unroll the towel until you have some lift but can lie comfortably.) Hold for about 10 easy, full breaths (or longer, if you're comfortable).

Caution: *Do not do this stretch during the second or third trimester of pregnancy or if you have spinal or neck disk problems. Don't let your head fall backward or the front of your throat overstretch. Reposition the towel a little lower on your spine or reduce the height of the rolled towel if your shoulders don't reach the ground comfortably.*

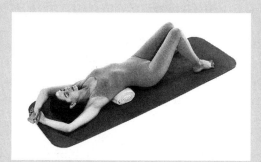

Take your arms over your head and, if your hands reach the ground comfortably, rest one palm in the other.

The second exercise is a gentle twist of the spine that stretches cramped muscles of the back, sides, and shoulders. It feels fantastic, not only after gardening but also after any activity where you've spent too much time hunching forward—sitting, driving, sewing, computing. You'll be amazed at how relaxing just a few minutes of breathing while in these positions can be.

Lie on your back, this time without the towel, with your feet flat on the floor and arms resting at your sides. Slowly lower your legs sideways to the right, toward the floor. Hold for 15 relaxing breaths, then bring your legs back up. Pause for several breaths, then repeat to the left. To come up without hurting your back or tensing your abdomen, roll onto one side, into the fetal position. Then use your hands to push your torso up, letting your head come up last.

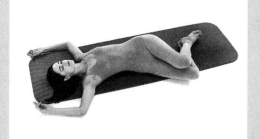

of our patients still use the tapes from our clinic 10 to 15 years later."

Classes in relaxation also are available. Check at your local hospital or look under "stress reduction" or "meditation instruction" in the Yellow Pages.

Be prepared to expect the unexpected. At a branch of Dr. Benson's Mind/Body Institute in Houston, for instance, the atmosphere is as casual as an aerobics class. In fact, when the instructor says, "Everyone get a mat," you might think that you should have worn your tights and cross-trainers.

The institute itself is a couple of carpeted rooms at the back of a nondescript office building, with treadmills and stairclimbers clustered in a corner. Not exactly the incense-filled room with contortionists for instructors that you might envision. "The casual atmosphere is intentional," Dr. Benson says. "People relate to it better."

But you can relax just as well at home with a guided-imagery tape. Whatever your approach, once you've relaxed for 10 to 20 minutes, count to three and slowly open your eyes.

Dr. Benson and other experts suggest an initial goal of one full relaxation session daily. Ideally, build a habit by unwinding each day at the same time. "You may find that if you do it right before bedtime, it's a good way to drift into sleep," says Margaret A. Caudill, M.D., Ph.D., co-director of the Arnold Pain Center at Beth Israel Deaconess Medical Center and author of *Managing Pain before It Manages You.* "Or you may find it a good way to start the day, with a clear mind."

Once you've made it routine, you can add impromptu sessions as pain arises, says Jim Spira, Ph.D., a licensed psychologist and director of the Institute for Health Psychology in San Diego. "It's such a simple technique that it can be practiced on airplanes, subways, and in the office. If you wake up in the middle of the night because of pain, you can get into a comfortable chair, practice your technique, and then return to bed."

You'll get even more out of your daily session if you take a break for a few seconds every hour to relax your jaw, breathe deeply, and loosen your tight shoulders, says Dr. Caudill. "By doing this, you won't have 24 hours worth of tension to dissipate at once."

A single session of these relaxation techniques can often relieve mild pain caused by something like a tension headache almost immediately, experts say. But don't expect more serious types of pain to go away quite so quickly. Studies suggest that you can expect arthritic, back, or other severe pain to lessen after about a month of regular relaxation sessions. It also takes that long for the benefits to start lasting all day, as your body changes its response to stress hormones. Before you realize it, you'll transform from a coiled snake to a lounging cat.

But unlike in animals, such languor in humans isn't inborn, Dr. Caudill says. "You have to practice constantly in the beginning so you develop a protection against the fight-or-flight response to stress."

Keep in mind, relaxation is not about wiping out your thoughts and feelings. It's about making room for calmness and peace in your life. "People think that deep relaxation is about trying to find a special switch in their minds that shuts things off or puts them in a 'special state.' But everyone's mind goes all over the place," says Dr. Kabat-Zinn. "We tell our patients that we are going to teach them how to be so relaxed that it is okay to be tense at times and to just experience that. Trying to make everything you don't like go away can be unrealistic and self-defeating."

With deep relaxation comes enhanced calmness. "You'll find a greater sense of self-confidence, knowing that you're more in charge of your life and pain," says Dr. Kabat-Zinn. "Deep relaxation isn't a magic pill you take, but a way of being."

Allergies

Usually, your immune system wages battle against potentially harmful invaders. But if you're one of the many Americans with allergies, your immune system becomes just a little too efficient, and that's when trouble can ensue.

Search and destroy. That is the main goal of your immune system, a complex network of specialized cells that is constantly on alert for viruses, bacteria, parasites, and other alien organisms. Its job, quite simply, is to get them before they get you.

But when your immune system takes aim against a harmless foreign substance like pollen, your body releases histamines and other chemicals that produce symptoms of an allergic response. Those symptoms can range from a little case of the sniffles to (less commonly) a full-blown, life-threatening, body-wide reaction called anaphylaxis, marked by breathing difficulties and a dangerous drop in blood pressure. Various foods, drugs, pollen, animal dander, dust mites, plants, or insect stings can spark allergic reactions.

Environmental pollution, food additives, and pesticides have combined to make people more allergically reactive than ever before, says Martha Howard, M.D., co-director of Wellness Associates, a Chicago-based family medical practice. "We treat more and more people with allergies these days. It's practically an epidemic."

Here's what alternative medicine has to offer for two of the most common types of allergy: hay fever and food allergies.

Hay Fever: Let Nature Cure

It's not caused by hay, and you don't get a fever when you have it. So precisely what is hay fever, anyway?

Sometimes described as the most common and annoying allergy around, hay fever affects around 40 million Americans, who suffer through it with sneezing, wheezing, runny noses, and itchy, watery eyes. There are two varieties: Seasonal hay fever occurs only when certain allergens, such as pollen, are airborne; perennial hay fever is a year-round allergy to things like animal dander and dust mites.

"Allergies to airborne irritants tend to run in families," says Lisa Meserole, doctor of naturopathy, research consultant, and faculty member in the botanical medicine department at Bastyr University of Naturopathic Medicine in Seattle.

The medical approach to managing hay fever often calls for taking antihistamines—over-the-counter or prescription medications that relieve symptoms by blocking the release of histamines, the substances responsible for hay fever symptoms. The problem is, antihistamines can (and often do) leave people feeling tired.

How to Hamstring Hay Fever

Thankfully, natural medicine offers some highly effective alternatives that, combined with basic avoidance tactics, may eliminate (or at least lessen) your need for fatigue-provoking drugs. Here are the experts' suggestions.

Move or adapt. "The classic recommendation for hay fever is to reduce your exposure as much as possible," says Dr. Meserole. "If you have a bad seasonal allergy—hay fever triggered by pollen, for example—and you can't move to another part of the country, then you have to eliminate pollen from the air that you breathe."

Dr. Meserole advises her patients to use air filters at home and in the office and to clean their home furnace vents regularly. (Conventional physicians often give the same advice.)

Give your immune system a hand. Supporting your general health helps your immune system fight off outside invaders, says Dr. Meserole. "So eat plenty of fruits and vegetables, be sure to exercise regularly, get enough sleep, and make sure to laugh heartily several times a day.

"When your immune system is stressed out from a poor diet, lack of sleep, or other problems, you can become apparently allergic to things that wouldn't normally cause you to react," says Dr. Meserole.

"And when you're really run-down and exhausted, your adrenal glands and the hormones that they secrete—epinephrine and norepinephrine—are affected. White blood cells fail to migrate properly, histamine release is off-balance, and as a result, your body mounts an ineffective and overreactive immune response to allergens," explains Dr. Howard.

Meditate hay fever into submission. Practicing meditation or yoga regularly can help turn hay fever around, says Dr. Meserole. "Both disciplines allow you to reach the ideal state of relaxation that makes it easier for your body to heal itself and ease allergic symptoms."

Key into C. "High doses of vitamin C alone, between 2 and 5 grams a day (2,000 to 5,000 milligrams in divided doses), will reduce hay fever symptoms in some people because vitamin C at these levels has an antihistamine action," says Dr. Meserole. "Though I've also seen it not work, it's totally safe, cheap, and readily available." (If you're prone to kidney stones, however, you shouldn't exceed 500 milligrams of vitamin C a day. Also, excess vitamin C above 1,200 milligrams a day may cause diarrhea in some people.)

Food Allergies: A Tough Riddle to Solve

When it comes to dealing with food allergies, the solutions are more complicated, mainly because reactions to food are so confusing, says Melvyn Werbach, M.D., assistant clinical professor of psychiatry at the

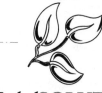

*Herbal*SOLUTION

Take the Sting Out of Allergies

Many people reach for antihistamines whenever they need hay fever relief. But a natural remedy—stinging nettles—is favored by experts in herbal medicine. Freeze-dried nettle leaves can bring dramatic relief if you have hay fever, according to Andrew Weil, M.D., professor of herbalism and director of the Program of Integrative Medicine at the University of Arizona College of Medicine, near Tucson, and author of *Spontaneous Healing.*

If you want to try out this herbal antihistamine, you can get various preparations in health food stores. "Use freeze-dried nettles in capsules, tinctures, or teas according to label directions," says Lisa Meserole, doctor of naturopathy, research consultant, and faculty member in the botanical medicine department at Bastyr University of Naturopathic Medicine in Seattle. She recommends that you try a small dose first since some people are sensitive to nettles.

Or try a preparation made from the roots, suggests James A. Duke, Ph.D., a retired U.S. Department of Agriculture botanist and author of *The Green Pharmacy.* "Every spring, visitors to my herb garden dig up roots from my nettle patch to treat their hay fever," says Dr. Duke. "For centuries, cultures around the world have used this herb to treat nasal and respiratory troubles."

University of California, Los Angeles, and author of *Nutritional Influences on Illness.*

Foods can cause two kinds of reactions in people who are sensitive. As with allergic reactions to airborne allergens like dust, one is a true allergic reaction to certain foods that cause specific symptoms, such as hives, watery eyes, sneezing, wheezing, and sinus congestion.

Seafood, especially shellfish, is among the foods that most commonly trigger allergic symptoms. Nuts are also villains, and some people have very severe reactions to them. (And peanuts, which are legumes, cause more allergy-related deaths than any other food.) Wheat, corn, milk, soy, and eggs have all been implicated as allergy-causers. And allergists have found that egg whites are even bigger troublemakers than the yolks.

The second kind of reaction—food sensitivity—isn't an allergy in the true sense of the word. That is, your body doesn't release histamines or other chemicals typically triggered by allergens. Food sensitivity causes a broad variety of less specific reactions.

"Severe food sensitivity can cause all kinds of problems, ranging from headaches and stomachaches to confusion and other vague complaints," says Dr. Werbach. Food sensitivity has been implicated in conditions as diverse as eczema, arthritis, colitis, ear infections, asthma, and glaucoma.

According to Dr. Werbach, the science of food sensitivity is advancing, and doctors are increasingly aware of the problem.

"We now know that partially broken down proteins can get into the immune system through the intestines," explains Dr. Werbach. "This tendency, called gut permeability, or leaky gut syndrome, can sensitize people to foods like milk and wheat."

Doctors have also discovered that food sensitivities can come and go, says Dr. Werbach. Eating certain foods frequently can sensitize you to them, he adds. "I remember one woman, for example, who was sensitive to cow's milk. So she stopped drinking cow's milk and started drinking goat's milk, but then she became sensitive to goat's milk. Now she's back to cow's milk again, and she's feeling just fine."

Ironically, some doctors believe that frequent cravings for a specific food might mean that you're sensitive to that food. Though no one knows exactly how common food allergies and food sensitivities are, Dr. Werbach estimates that perhaps 3 percent of us have classic allergic reactions to specific foods, and he suspects that many more of us may be food-sensitive, at least some of the time.

Zeroing In on the Foods That Bother You

Blood and skin tests for allergies aren't always reliable, says Dr. Werbach. So if you suspect that you're reacting to something that you're eating, he suggests that you try an elimination diet instead. Here's how.

Avoid foods that you eat more than twice a week. This usually includes wheat, dairy products, yeast, and corn, says Dr. Werbach. You'll have to become a devoted label-reader during that time and stay away from bakery items and packaged foods that contain these ingredients.

Give it a couple of weeks. Problems such as headaches will clear up within a few days if the eliminated food is to blame. Some symptoms, such as joint pain, could take much longer to fade. So one to two weeks of elimination is optimal to figure out what's causing most problems, says Dr. Werbach.

If in doubt, leave it out. To make sure that you're not getting ingredients that you're trying to avoid, you may have to do more than read ingredient lists closely. Sometimes those lists are vague or incomplete, or they have chemical names that aren't familiar to you. If you don't know exactly what's in a particular food, avoid it, advises Dr. Werbach.

Reintroduce foods slowly. Once you've started to feel better, add back the eliminated foods one at a time, every three days, to pinpoint the one that troubles you, says Dr. Werbach.

Keep track. Write down exactly what you eat and when. Note symptoms, too, and any changes. Rate symptoms on a scale of 1 to 10 and compare them over time. This log should further help you identify (and avoid) foods that cause problems.

Stay away from the prime culprits. Once you've pinned down problem foods, avoid them, says Dr. Werbach.

Arthritis

If you thought the last word on arthritis was, "Pop painkillers and suffer," you haven't been talking to the right sources. New research brings hope that what you eat can ease your pain.

Where two bones come together, you have a joint. And if the joint is healthy, the ends of those bones should be covered with a resilient padding—called cartilage—that reduces friction and absorbs shock as you move about. But nearly 16 million Americans have to deal with one kind of arthritis—called osteoarthritis—that causes pain and swelling when the cartilage in certain joints begins to deteriorate. In fact, sometimes that cartilage diminishes so much that it's entirely worn away. Why this happens is still uncertain, though heredity is thought to be part of the cause.

The outcome, unfortunately, is less uncertain. When poorly padded bones rub together, pain results. Joints affected most by osteoarthritis seem to be hands, hips, and knees—usually resulting in the most disabling form of osteoarthritis. Sometimes inflammation and swelling accompany the pain. Another common consequence is stiffness and loss of mobility, as people with osteoarthritis avoid activity in an attempt to avoid the hurt.

Taking the Burden Off

Now, there's growing confidence among osteoarthritis experts about the most effective dietary strategy to soothe your joints. If you're beyond a healthy weight (as many people with osteoarthritis are), try losing a few pounds, especially through a combination of diet and exercise.

Look what happened to 48 overweight postmenopausal women with osteoarthritis of the knees who participated in a diet-exercise trial at the University of Maryland School of Medicine in College Park. After six months of walking on a treadmill three times a week (up to 45 minutes per session) and following a reduced-calorie, low-fat diet, the women lost an average of 15½ pounds each.

And here's the key payoff: They had much less knee pain. Using a reliable measure called the WOMAC pain score, 40 percent of the women reported only half as much pain. A third of the women experienced a 50 percent improvement in functions such as walking up stairs and getting in and out of cars. And compared with the beginning of the study, on average, the women walked 12 percent farther on a 6-minute walking test.

There is also evidence that losing even less weight may be enough to relieve pain. In a study at Bowman Gray School of Medicine of Wake Forest University in Winston-Salem, North Carolina, men and women over age 60 with osteoarthritis of the knees lost an average of 19 pounds over six months with a diet-and-exercise combo. Again, pain declined and performance improved. "But some people who lost only 10 pounds experienced as much improvement in pain and disability as those who lost much more," says Walter Ettinger, M.D., an osteoarthritis researcher and professor of internal medicine at Bowman Gray.

Why does losing just a few pounds seem to help so much? Rheumatologist Marc Hochberg, M.D., who headed the University of Maryland study, explains it this way: When you walk, with each step, your knee absorbs a force equal to about three times your body weight. So losing even 10 pounds actually relieves each knee of more like a 30-pound load with every stride.

Can losing weight help in more ways than reducing pressure? Maybe. "It's well-known that being overweight raises the risk of getting osteoarthritis in the first place. But why do obese women get more osteoarthritis of the hand, an area that wouldn't be stressed from being overweight?" asks researcher David Felson, M.D., of Boston University School of Medicine. "Perhaps," he suggests, "obesity in itself exerts some metabolic influence on bone and cartilage."

The bottom line is, if you're overweight and have osteoarthritis, lose at least 10 pounds. Dr. Hochberg stresses that it's critical to both exercise and cut calories to lose weight. "Studies show that the combination is more effective for losing weight. Plus, we know that sticking with exercise helps keep weight off

Can You B Happy?

Could two B vitamins—B_{12} and folic acid—work better than drugs do on your osteoarthritis? That's what one small yet promising study hints. Researcher Margaret Flynn, R.D., Ph.D., professor emeritus at the University of Missouri in Columbia, gathered a group of 26 patients with osteoarthritis of the hand and took them off all nonsteroidal anti-inflammatory drugs for pain.

Patients were allowed the milder over-the-counter medicine acetaminophen, as needed. Dr. Flynn found that patients taking 20 micrograms of vitamin B_{12} plus 6,400 micrograms of folic acid for two months had the same grip strength but fewer tender joints compared with when they started the study and compared with when they took just folic acid or a placebo for two months. Some patients on the combination of B_{12} and folic acid were able to decrease their acetaminophen dosage.

To evaluate this very preliminary finding, we went to Ronenn Roubenoff, M.D., a rheumatologist and nutritionist at Tufts University in Medford, Massachusetts. He made several points.

• Though intriguing and worth following up, until other studies repeat these results, vitamin B_{12} plus folic acid is not recognized as a treatment for osteoarthritis.

for the long haul." (Before starting an exercise program, check with your doctor to find out how much exercise is safe for you.)

Slow Osteoarthritis with a Little C

For 10 years researchers have kept track of 640 residents of Framingham, Massachusetts, who have osteoarthritis, including recording what they ate. It turns out that those getting the most vitamin C had a threefold reduction in osteoarthritis progression—meaning that they lost less knee cartilage over time—compared with those getting the least vitamin C.

"Vitamin C may help because it plays a role in making collagen, a material necessary for repairing cartilage," says Boston University's Tim McAlindon, M.D., lead researcher of the study. He notes that people getting the middle range of vitamin C daily (about 150 to 175 milligrams—

- The amounts of vitamin B_{12} and folic acid (though far above Daily Value levels) are within the safe range as long as both vitamins are taken together. Taking this much folic acid alone could mask a serious deficiency of B_{12} in some older people.
- People considering vitamin B_{12} and folic acid should check with their doctors first. One osteoarthritis patient who decided to give B_{12} and folic acid a try was Judy Miles, M.D., Ph.D., a 46-year-old physician who is director of medical genetics at the University of Missouri School of Medicine. "I was getting incapacitated from osteoarthritis of the hands, waking up at least twice a night to take acetaminophen," she recounts. "And I knew that trying B_{12} and folic acid at these levels wasn't going to hurt me."

Gradually, on 20 micrograms of B_{12} plus 6,000 micrograms of folic acid daily, Dr. Miles found her need for acetaminophen tablets dropping. In two months she went from 10 a day to none—a sign of dramatic reduction in pain, she says.

Dr. Miles agrees that her experience in no way constitutes scientific proof that the B_{12}-plus-folic-acid combination works against osteoarthritis pain (her story is what's called anecdotal evidence), and that there could be other explanations for her relief. But this does add to the hope that researchers will follow up this tantalizing lead with more studies.

*Herbal*SOLUTION

Brew for Arthritis Relief

A wide variety of herbs—all brewed in a simmering broth—can help relieve arthritis pain, according to James A. Duke, a retired U.S. Department of Agriculture botanist and author of *The Green Pharmacy*. He recommends using some or all of the following ingredients, adjusting the proportion of ingredients to suit your taste.

2	**cups water**
4	**parts burdock**
4	**parts dandelion**
4	**parts parsley**
4	**parts turmeric**
4	**parts watercress**
2	**parts celery seed**
2	**parts garlic**
2	**parts ginger**
2	**parts oregano**
1	**part each of sweet red peppers, black pepper, horseradish, juniper, lemongrass, sarsaparilla, thyme, valerian, white mustard, and willow bark**

Add the herbs to the water, and bring to a boil. Reduce the heat and simmer for a few minutes.

an amount easy to get from food) had the same reduced risk of osteoarthritis progression as those taking the most vitamin C (430 to 500 milligrams). His conclusion? It might not be the vitamin C alone that's helping with the repair work, but other healing compounds in foods that contain C. So you can't count on a vitamin C supplement alone; be sure to eat the foods that contain vitamin C.

The bottom line is that you should eat at least five servings of fruits and vegetables daily, making sure to include rich sources of vitamin C. If you live east of the Mississippi River, look for an unexpected source of vitamin C in specially bred fresh pineapple called Del Monte Gold. One cup of Del Monte Gold pineapple (about two slices) has 60 milligrams of vitamin C, compared with 15 milligrams for regular pineapple. As a delicious bonus, Del Monte Gold pineapple tastes extra sweet, too. See "Serving Up Vitamin C" for top sources.

A Dose of D Douses Osteoarthritis

Another finding from the Framingham study offers one more potential clue to slowing osteoarthritis with diet: getting at least 360 international units (IU) of vitamin D a day. People with vitamin D intakes lower than this level were about three times more likely to have progression of knee osteoarthritis.

Serving Up Vitamin C

Here's a list of fruits and vegetables that are rich sources of vitamin C.

Food	Vitamin C (mg.)
1 guava	165
1 sweet red pepper	141
1 cup fresh-squeezed orange juice	124
1 cup cranberry juice cocktail	108
1 cup orange juice from concentrate	97
1 cup papaya	87
1 cup strawberries	85
1 cup grapefruit juice from concentrate	83
1 cup raw broccoli florets	82
1 kiwifruit	75
1 orange	70
1 cup cantaloupe cubes	68
1 green pepper	66
1 cup pineapple	60
1 mango	57
1 cup raw cauliflower florets	46
1/2 grapefruit	41

How might vitamin D help slow osteoarthritis? It is known to play a role in keeping bones healthy. Dr. McAlindon notes that once osteoarthritis breaks down cartilage in a joint, the underlying bone is subjected to greater stress. Low levels of vitamin D may impair the ability of bone to respond to this increased wear and tear.

One way to ensure that you consume enough vitamin D per day is to look for a multivitamin with 400 IU (equal to 100 percent of the Daily Value, or DV). The only other substantial dietary sources of vitamin D include the following: 1 cup of any type of milk has 100 IU (25 percent of the DV); ⅓ cup of nonfat dry milk has 100 IU; and some breakfast cereals are fortified with 40 IU per serving (10 percent of the DV). Experts recommend getting no more than 600 IU of vitamin D daily.

Though we'll need more studies to confirm the benefits of losing weight and especially of getting enough of vitamins C and D, why wait to start? We already know that these measures boost your health in plenty of other ways. But suffering less osteoarthritis pain—now and years down the road—could be your most welcome reward of all.

Back Pain

Rocket scientists have finally perfected the office chair. But there are plenty of less costly ways to keep back pain at bay.

At last, space-age science has finally been applied to a matter of utmost importance: the comfortable cradling of your back and lower posterior. There is actually something called the Zero Gravity K-Series chair, which is designed to put an end to the kind of back pain caused by poor office furnishings that is suffered by thousands of seated workers throughout the United States.

By studying zero-gravity data collected during both the NASA Skylab and space-shuttle missions, BodyBilt Seating has determined that a free-floating body will assume a 128-degree trunk-to-thigh ratio, which

Good Sex with a Bad Back

When you have a bad back and you're making love, your first concern is to avoid arching backward, which places great stress on the joints of the lower (lumbar) spine. You also want to avoid lying flat. Bent knees and flexed hips, on the other hand, relax the psoas muscles that extend from the front of the lumbar spine to below the hip joints, and that, in turn, takes pressure off your lower back.

As you've probably just figured out, the standard missionary position is a no-go. Augustus A. White III, M.D., doctor of medical science and professor of orthopedic surgery at Harvard Medical School, recommends the following back-safe sex positions, no matter which partner has the back problem.

1. The classic "spoons" position: Both partners lie on their sides, knees bent, man behind the woman. Nobody bears any body weight.
2. Man on his back, his upper torso supported by pillows if he has a bad back: The woman straddles him; her knees are bent, and she's facing him with her back bent forward, the weight of her upper torso supported by her arms.
3. Same as above (in number 2), but with the woman facing away from the man and her hands on his knees.
4. In a hot tub: The man is in a sitting position, and the woman faces him while sitting on his thighs. Warmth and buoyancy take things from there.
5. Woman on her back, her knees bent and her upper torso supported by pillows: The man kneels, supporting her thighs with his thighs and arms.

provides the best musculoskeletal alignment. Not only does their chair allow the body to achieve this slightly reclined posture without actually slumping but a 10-point posture-control system also allows users to tailor their comfort in a way that's just not possible with the average office chairs in most workplaces today. In fact, so serious is BodyBilt that they include an owner's manual on a computer disk with each chair.

Now the bad news. The Zero Gravity K-Series starts at around $895, leaving you to ask yourself one very important question: Which is

Stretch for a Better Back

Owners of cranky backs know that it can take as little as a reach for a shoelace to push a sensitive back over the brink into spasm. And we know that in the heat of the moment, ice is the key. But do you know what to do when the pain subsides? If you're smart, you don't just say "thank goodness" and go back to life as usual. You do what helps prevent further attacks: You stretch.

These stretches don't target your back; they're aimed at your hamstrings, the muscles that run from the pelvis down the backs of the thighs to the knees. They're one of the most common contributors to lower-back pain. When they get tight, they shorten and tilt the pelvis backward, restricting its movement.

"Then, when you bend forward at the hips, your pelvis can't tilt forward with you," says Edward Laskowski, M.D., co-director of the sports medicine center at the Mayo Clinic in Rochester, Minnesota. "This causes increased stress on the lower back." If it gets too stressed, the muscles in the area spasm. The spasm is a protective response to initial injury and helps to prevent further damage.

The backward tilting of the pelvis also flattens the natural curve of the lower back. "The gentle curves in the back are what distribute a load evenly along the spine and prevent excess stress to any one spot," says Dr. Laskowski. "Taking the curve out of the lower back makes the muscles work extra hard and puts pressure on spinal disks."

Unless you stretch regularly, your hamstrings are bound to be tight, says John Friend, certified Iyengar yoga instructor and creator of the video *Yoga: Alignment and Form*. Both activity and inactivity make them shorten. The reclining stretch shown here lets you relax on the floor while you isolate and stretch just the hamstring muscles.

"The longer your hamstrings are, the more freedom of movement your pelvis will have," says Friend. "That takes undue pressure off the lower back." Try this hamstring stretch at least once a day and do it five days a week, he suggests. Before you start, have a belt and a pillow handy.

more uncomfortable, your current office chair or the unemployment line you may be standing in after you demand that your boss provide you with one of these?

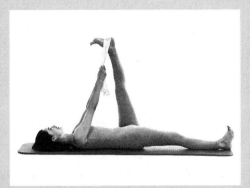

Lie down on your back. Support your head with a pillow. Bring your feet together so that your toes and knees point toward the ceiling. On an exhalation, draw your left knee in to your chest. Wrap a towel or belt around your left foot, holding one end in each hand. Slowly extend your foot and leg up, bending the knee slightly. Only draw your left leg as far toward your chest as you can while keeping it as straight as possible and keeping your right thigh pressing down. Don't bounce. Hold for 30 seconds, repeating two times on each side, then unloop the towel or belt from your foot and return your leg to the floor. Do the same with the other leg, then repeat twice, alternating legs.

Helpful hint: Don't just yank your left leg toward your chest. Bending your knee reduces the stretch to the hamstring. Make sure that your leg stays straight, even if you have to lower it toward the floor. At the point where you can keep your knee straight and still feel the stretch, stop and hold for 30 seconds. To make the stretch uniform along the entire length of the hamstring, press your left thighbone backward toward your hamstring even as you hold your foot steady with the belt.

Making your feet active instead of floppy will give you a better stretch in your legs. To do it, strongly press away from your hips through your heel. Press also through the ball of your foot, particularly the mound under the big toe. Spread your toes apart and draw them back toward your head.

Luckily, there's a lot that you can do to rectify the back-pain potential of the office chair that you currently perch on. The fine art of comfortable sitting, while simple enough, does require a little thought, a little

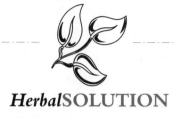

*Herbal*SOLUTION

These Wondrous Cures
Ease Back Pain

For occasional back pain, there are a number of herbal alternatives that can prove helpful.

- Willow (*Salix,* various species) and other forms of "natural aspirin." Aspirin originally came from compounds known as salicylates that occur naturally in willow bark, meadowsweet, milkwort, and wintergreen. Any of these herbs can be made into pain-relieving teas, says James A. Duke, Ph.D., a retired U.S. Department of Agriculture botanist and author of *The Green Pharmacy*.

  Many salicylate-rich plants also contain methyl salicylate, an aspirin-like compound with a particularly pleasing smell. One is wintergreen. Another is birch bark, once used by Native Americans to make a tea that they drank or applied externally to treat lower-back pain. Dr. Duke occasionally makes such teas by throwing a handful of birch bark, wintergreen, or milkwort into a cup or two of boiling water and letting it steep for about 10 minutes.

- Oil of wintergreen (*Gaultheria procumbens*). This is high in methyl salicylate and serves as a good pain reliever for external use, Dr.

planning, and adherence to a few rules. Put these things into play, and you may never need to find out whether the boss thinks you're worth $895 . . . plus tax.

A Room with a Chair

The most crucial thing you need to realize is that no chair is an island. In other words, your office chair is meant to be used in the context of your whole work environment. Here often lies the problem.

"The best chair in the world isn't going to help you if you have a

Duke says. It may be applied during massage.

Caution: Make sure that you keep oil of wintergreen out of children's reach. It has a tempting aroma, but ingesting even a little can prove fatal.

- Red pepper (*Capsicum annuum*). This contains a marvelous pain-relieving chemical—capsaicin—that is so potent that a tiny amount provides the active ingredient in some powerful pharmaceutical topical analgesics. (Zostix and Axsain contain only 0.025 percent capsaicin.)

At this point researchers aren't sure whether red pepper's effectiveness is due to capsaicin's ability to interfere with pain perception, its ability to trigger the release of the body's own pain-relieving endorphins, its salicylates, or all three.

You can buy a commercial cream containing capsaicin and use that. Outside the United States, however, people simply use red pepper. You can, too, for considerable savings. A hot pepper costs a few cents, while capsaicin costs a few dollars.

You can mash a red pepper and rub it directly on the painful area, Dr. Duke says. You can also take any white skin cream that you have on hand—cold cream will do—and mix in enough red pepper to turn it pink. Remember to wash off all traces of red pepper before you put your fingers near your face. You don't want to get this stuff in your eyes.

miserable work environment," says Malcolm H. Pope, Ph.D., doctor of medical science, of the Spinal Research Center at the University of Iowa in Iowa City.

"The first thing that you really want to do is assess your desk area to see how much it forces you to twist, turn, hunch, and crane in uncomfortable ways." If you write or read at your desk, you may want to consider several well-placed pieces of plywood to set your work surface up at a 35-degree tilt toward you. "This will immediately put your neck and lumbar spine in a better position so that you are not craning forward just to see what it is that you are working on," says Dr. Pope.

And if you're using a computer, placement is equally important. "The computer monitor should be at a level that you can easily view without having to look up or having to look down," says Dr. Pope. "In other words, you want to try to keep your head over your shoulders rather than having it sink between them as you try to look down at the terminal. Meanwhile, the keyboard should be close enough so that you don't find yourself having to lean forward to reach it in order to type."

Location, Location, Location

Placement plays a role in where you keep your files and other work tools as well. "One thing that will put a lot of stress on your back is constantly reaching up or down for things that you need," says Jeffrey Young, M.D., assistant professor of physical medicine and rehabilitation at Northwestern University Medical School in Chicago. "My personal rule is to never put things in the lowest desk drawers if I'm going to be using them frequently. Instead, I'll keep these kinds of items in one of the top drawers, allowing me the ability to reach for them without actually having to lean down. And if I do have to get something from a lower desk drawer, I'll get out of my chair first."

Speaking of getting out of the chair, do it, and do it frequently. "No matter how good a chair may be, it's not meant to be sat in constantly," says Dr. Pope. "Your best protection against back pain is to make a point of getting out of your chair and moving at least once an hour."

Bone Up on Sitting Right

Okay, so bad chairs happen to good people. But how you sit in that chair can make a world of difference. The fact is, most people really aren't all that sure how to sit well or even how to use some of the simple adjustments that most modern office chairs offer. Here's what you can do.

Let your feet touch the floor. If your feet are dangling, your thighs are bearing too much weight. "You can lower the actual height of the seat," says Dr. Young. "But if that puts you in a position where your desk is too high, try resting your feet on a small footstool." When sitting properly, your knee joints should form a nice 90-degree angle. "Generally, if a chair is hitting you right, you won't even realize that your feet are on the floor because the pressure is so evenly distributed over your feet, legs, and butt," says Dr. Young.

Extend your knees 2 to 3 inches past the edge of the chair. "If your knees are draped right over the lip of the chair, you may run into some circulatory problems," cautions Dr. Pope. "If the depth of the chair is adjustable, you might start by moving the back piece in a couple of inches so that you are sitting a little more forward in the seat. If it isn't adjustable, try a pillow behind you, as long as it doesn't make you feel uncomfortable."

Don't sit like a cadet. "Sit up straight" may not be the best advice your mother ever gave you, according to Dr. Pope. "The imperative here is to try to reduce the amount of stress on the disks, and studies show that pressure really starts to decrease when your back is not perfectly vertical and ramrod straight."

So rather than forming a perfect "L" with your body, try leaning back in the chair a bit . . . but no slumping.

Maintain good lumbar support. Your lumbar region is that curvature of your lower back, which is easily felt while standing up but seems to disappear when you sit down. You don't want it to disappear.

"One way to support the lumbar region is to adjust the back of your chair," says Dr. Young. "If you have one of those secretarial seats that is open-backed near the bottom, adjust the backrest so that the bottom of it squares with the small of your back and the top at least catches the bottom of your shoulder blades." And if the back of your seat is not adjustable, a small rolled-up towel placed behind the small of your back helps support this area nicely.

Cholesterol

Keeping your arteries clean and lean is easier than you think. In this chapter by former U.S. surgeon general Joycelyn Elders, M.D., you'll discover plenty of simple tricks to skim cholesterol from your diet.

Cholesterol—a fancy word for fat that has changed its chemical composition a bit in the body—does a lot more than just clog a few arteries. When cholesterol is gumming up the works, it becomes difficult or impossible for your body to pump oxygen-rich blood efficiently from one organ to another, and all sorts of trouble comes to pass.

A clogged circulatory system is an invitation to high blood pressure, several types of heart disease, stroke, and even increased complications from conditions such as diabetes. The great news, however, is that most people have almost complete control over their cholesterol levels. All it

Exercise Can Put Cholesterol Crunch in High Gear

Low-fat. Low-fat. Low-fat. It's been your mantra for months now. And while your belt has tightened a notch, your cholesterol levels haven't dipped as much as you'd like them to. Research suggests that if you want to significantly influence cholesterol in your kitchen, you should probably move your treadmill in there, too. Of course, watching what you eat can certainly curb cholesterol levels that have been speeding skyward. But to send them tumbling even farther, try adding exercise to your routine.

In a study of 377 men and women with moderately high low-density lipoprotein (LDL), or bad, cholesterol and moderately low amounts of high-density lipoprotein (HDL), or good, cholesterol, Stanford University researchers in Palo Alto, California, saw that people who added a workout to a low-fat eating plan for a year sent LDL cholesterol down about two times as much as did people who tried to eat their way to good health without exercise.

Women who added exercise to smart eating lowered their LDL almost 12 milligrams per deciliter (mg/dl) more than people who did nothing. Men who did the same saw LDL drop by about 15 mg/dl over people whose diets and exercise habits didn't change. Good eating alone (less than 25 percent of calories from fat) changed LDL only about 5 to 6 mg/dl for men and women. Exercise alone did next to nothing to nudge cholesterol out of the high zone in this study.

"This demonstrates that exercise is not only important for HDL cholesterol, which is where exercise has been thought to have a role, but that exercise is also very important for managing LDL cholesterol. Previously, people have focused only on diet to manage this," says Stanford

takes is a bit of knowledge and a little work.

To beat cholesterol, it helps to understand it. First, your arteries begin to collect fatty deposits during childhood. So the best way to stay healthy is to start out in life with a low-fat, high-fiber diet. If you missed that opportunity, the next step is to take charge of your diet as an adult.

The goal is not to eliminate cholesterol from your body—because you need a moderate amount of it for proper biochemical functioning—

study author Marcia Stefanick, Ph.D.

Exercise is thought to influence LDL by helping people lose abdominal fat, says study leader Peter Wood, D.Sc., Ph.D., associate director of the university's Center for Research in Disease Prevention. Abdominal fat is a problem, one theory goes, because the blood circulating through it drains right into the liver. The liver, receiving fat-laden blood, turns around and manufactures fat molecules like LDL. But when fat in the abdomen is reduced, the blood-fat mill in your liver might have fewer raw materials with which to create damaging LDL.

Another possible way that adding exercise to your smart-eating plan could curb high LDL is through weight loss. Men doing the dynamic exercise-and-diet duo lost more weight than did men who did the diet or exercise programs alone (and being at ideal weight has long been linked to lower LDL). Why women who added exercise to diet didn't see drops in weight is a puzzle for future research to sort out. But even at a steady weight, they saw beneficial LDL drops.

Exercisers in this study worked out for 45 minutes three times a week. A different study, from Barcelona, Spain, sheds light on how hard you may want to push yourself to better your cholesterol profile. This study looked at the HDL side of the cholesterol equation. Of 537 men studied, those who worked out for 15 minutes at a calorie-burning rate of 420 per hour had HDL levels about 2 mg/dl higher than those who worked out at a more moderate rate. Work out longer, get more benefits. The equation goes like this: For every 100 calories burned at that 420 calorie-per-hour pace, HDL was 2 mg/dl higher. That pace is equal to treadmill walking at a little more than 4 miles per hour or bicycling at 10 miles per hour. The men who upped the intensity to 9 calories a minute, or 540 calories per hour (a 5-mile-per-hour walk) saw their total cholesterol levels slip, too.

but to balance good and bad cholesterol and keep total cholesterol under control. The good stuff is high-density lipoprotein (HDL) cholesterol; the bad stuff is low-density lipoprotein (LDL) cholesterol. They've earned their names because high levels of HDL correlate with low levels of coronary heart disease, and high levels of LDL have been shown to increase levels of heart disease.

The other thing that you need to know is what level you are looking for. Healthy rates differ for some people based on age and other factors, but generally a total cholesterol level of 200 milligrams per deciliter (mg/dl) or below is best; 200 to 239 mg/dl is borderline and heading for trouble; and 240 mg/dl and above is high, and you need to get it under control.

Here are 20 tips from the Food and Drug Administration to help you make sure that you keep your numbers in check.

1. Use soft, tub-style margarine, which is higher in polyunsaturated (healthy) fats than hard stick margarine.
2. Use skim, low-fat (1%), or nonfat milk and stick with low-fat dairy products.
3. Buy lean cuts of meat, such as beef round and pork tenderloin, and trim away all visible fat.
4. Choose food-preparation methods that add little or no fat. For example, broil, bake, or roast meat, fish, and poultry instead of pan-frying or deep-fat frying. Try baked potatoes instead of french fries. Keep meats moist and add flavor by basting with broth or with lemon or tomato juice.
5. Season vegetables with herbs or spices instead of butter or margarine.
6. Make sure that you eat plenty of fish, poultry (without the skin), and dried peas and beans. All of these are better sources of protein than red meat.
7. Develop a taste for low-fat or fat-free lunchmeats and hot dogs instead of the high-fat varieties.
8. Use low-fat or nonfat plain yogurt as a substitute for sour cream in salad dressings and dips.
9. Dig into delicious, creamy sherbet, ice milk, sorbet, low-fat ice cream, or nonfat frozen yogurt instead of premium ice cream.
10. Try a savory egg-white omelet. Toss a few herbs and a little black pepper with egg whites (you might even add a little nonfat cheese).

*Herbal*SOLUTION

Let These Remedies Sink High Cholesterol

Along with getting adequate fiber from the foods you eat, there are also a number of individual foods and herbs that can prove helpful in taming cholesterol, says James A. Duke, Ph.D., a retired U.S. Department of Agriculture botanist and author of *The Green Pharmacy*.

- Garlic (*Allium sativum*) and onion (*Allium cepa*). Many studies show that the equivalent of one clove of garlic a day or half an onion lowers total cholesterol levels 10 to 15 percent in most people, Dr. Duke says. In one study people given 800 milligrams of garlic daily (about one clove) experienced lower cholesterol levels, plus lower blood pressure. Garlic is an approved remedy in Europe for cardiovascular conditions, especially high cholesterol, Dr. Duke says.

  In another study 2 to 3 tablespoons of onion oil a day helped lower cholesterol in about half of people with moderately high cholesterol. Their blood cholesterol levels fell 7 to 33 percent when they were taking onion oil, according to Dr. Duke.

- Ginger (*Zingiber officinale*). Many studies show that ginger helps lower cholesterol. Why not add some ginger to spice up other cholesterol-lowering foods? Dr. Duke asks.

- Fenugreek (*Trigonella foenum-graecum*). Fenugreek is rich in a soothing fiber called mucilage, Dr. Duke says. This herb's cholesterol-lowering activity has been demonstrated in laboratory experiments with animals and also demonstrated in humans.

If you must have the yolk, have one and discard the others. In recipes, substitute a teaspoon of polyunsaturated oil for each yolk you take out.

11. Reduce the amount of fat in recipes by a third to a half. If you use commercial cake mixes, for example, buy those that have you add

the fat or oil. Then use polyunsaturated oil (such as sunflower oil) and reduce the amount by a third while increasing the water. For example, if the recipe you are using calls for 3 tablespoons of oil, use only 2, then add an extra tablespoon of water.

12. Cut down on baked goods made with lard, coconut oil, palm-kernel oil, or shortening as well as those deep-fried in fat, such as doughnuts and crullers. Try bagels instead.

13. Serve single-crust (open-faced) pies instead of those with a top crust.

14. Use herbs or herb-flavored croutons instead of high-fat dressings or oil to flavor salads.

15. Make your own dessert toppings with nonfat dried milk or use low-fat yogurt or fresh fruit.

16. Try out part-skim or nonfat mozzarella and ricotta cheese in your favorite Italian recipes. Be sure to check the label for the fat content of the varieties that claim to be low-fat.

17. Make your own breading with ordinary bread crumbs. Store-bought bread crumbs usually have hydrogenated oils added for texture and flavor. Use your homemade crumbs to coat foods like meats or fish, then dip them in skim milk mixed with an egg white,

Love to Bake? Lose the Yolks

You don't have to forgo baking—or eating—your favorite cakes, cookies, and muffins because you're cutting back on cholesterol-laden eggs. Here's how to bake yolk-free treats.

Baking with egg whites. Not using egg yolks won't significantly affect the texture of baked goods, says Evelyn Tribole, R.D., a dietitian in Beverly Hills, California, and author of *Healthy Homestyle Cooking*. In fact, you probably won't notice the difference, she says. She recommends substituting two beaten egg whites for each whole egg.

If you're baking a product that calls for three or four whole eggs, however, substituting that many egg whites may create too much liquid. In that case you may want to use an egg substitute.

Baking with egg substitute. Some experts suggest replacing each whole egg with ¼ cup of egg substitute. But you can use more or less of this product to suit your taste.

dust on a little paprika, and oven-bake them to a crisp golden brown.

18. Use a nonstick pan coated with a vegetable-oil spray such as Pam—in place of butter, margarine, or oil—when sautéing foods.

19. Coat popcorn lightly with a vegetable-oil spray, then sprinkle with chili powder, onion powder, or cinnamon instead of cooking in oil and seasoning with butter and salt.

20. Check food labels carefully for hidden cholesterol and saturated fat. Look for the following terms: egg and egg-yolk solids; whole-milk solids; palm, palm-kernel, and coconut oils; milk chocolate; shortening; hydrogenated or hardened oils; lard; butter; beef fat; and suet. Limit your intake of any foods that contain these ingredients.

Eat, be healthy, and enjoy!

Colds and Flu

If cold and flu viruses seem to have a knack for finding you, take heart. There's plenty you can do to prevent one of these bugs from knocking you off kilter.

In the never-ending cold wars, germs always seem to get the best of us. And there is a good reason why: Cold and flu viruses are everywhere. These ubiquitous little critters are hardy travelers, hitching rides from one host to another at office parties, shopping malls, and skating rinks. Little wonder then that colds and flu are among the most common causes of illness worldwide. Each year in the United States alone, they cause 23 million days of missed work.

Even though most of us gradually develop antibodies to these pests, a typical adult still gets three or four colds a year. In addition, about one in four Americans gets knocked down by the flu annually.

But there are ample ways to bolster your natural defenses and outflank these cagey little creatures. Here's a look at what the top experts suggest.

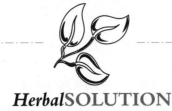

*Herbal*SOLUTION

Herbs Are Potent Allies during Cold and Flu Season

Quite a few herbs can help boost your immune system's cold-fighting power, according to James A. Duke, Ph.D., a retired U.S. Department of Agriculture botanist and author of *The Green Pharmacy*. Here's a sampling.

- Echinacea (*Echinacea angustifolia* and *E. purpurea*). This herb (pronounced ek-ih-NAY-see-uh)—a purple member of the daisy family—has antiviral properties, meaning that it bolsters immune systems to attack cold viruses and may help keep cold symptoms from blossoming. "Based on what we know so far, echinacea seems to work. But more clinical trials are needed to support claims of its effectiveness," says Varro E. Tyler, Ph.D., Sc.D, former professor of pharmacognosy at Purdue University in West Lafayette, Indiana, and author of *The New Honest Herbal* and *Herbs of Choice*. He recommends the liquid extract, or tincture, available in health food stores. Look for two things on the label: first, that the extract comes from either *E. angustifolia* or *E. purpurea* and second, that the preparation is standardized. Follow dosage directions carefully, since products can vary in their concentrations. Discontinue use as soon as symptoms disappear, since echinacea loses its effectiveness when taken for prolonged

Get vaccinated. Among folks officially recommended for flu shots are high-risk individuals, who include people age 65 and over, those with chronic health or respiratory problems, including children with asthma, and those with weak immune systems. But a study of 849 people conducted by Kristin Nichol, M.D., at the Veterans Affairs Medical Center in Minneapolis, shows that healthy, working adults may benefit, too. The half of the group who received real vaccine shots had 25 percent fewer upper respiratory illnesses, 43 percent fewer sick days from work due to respira-

periods. While side effects are seldom seen, if you are allergic to plants in the daisy family, taking echinacea could cause a runny nose and watery eyes, Dr. Tyler says.

- Garlic (*Allium sativum*). Eat enough garlic, and most people, along with their cold germs, will stay away from you. (Just joking.) There really are some excellent reasons to use this herb to prevent colds and flu. Garlic contains several helpful compounds, including allicin, one of the plant kingdom's most potent, broad-spectrum antibiotics, Dr. Duke says.

  As anyone who has ever had garlic breath knows, this herb's aromatic compounds are readily released from the lungs and respiratory tract, putting garlic's active ingredients right where they can be most effective against cold viruses.

- Ginger (*Zingiber officinale*). Pouring a cup of hot water onto a couple tablespoons of fresh, shredded ginger really makes a lot of sense as a cold treatment. That's because this herb contains nearly a dozen antiviral compounds, Dr. Duke says.

  Scientists have isolated several chemicals (sesquiterpenes) in ginger that have specific effects against the most common family of cold viruses, the rhinoviruses. Some of these chemicals are remarkably potent in their anti-rhinovirus effects.

  Still other constituents in ginger—gingerols and shogaols—help relieve cold symptoms because they reduce pain and fever, suppress cough, and have a mild sedative effect that encourages rest, Dr. Duke says.

tory illness, and 44 percent fewer doctor visits for upper respiratory illness than those who got placebo shots.

Scrub-a-dub. Cold and flu viruses are often spread by hand-to-mouth or hand-to-eye contact. Washing your hands several times a day will lessen the chances of secondary bacterial infections. In public, avoid drying your hands on shared cloth towels in public restrooms. Instead, keep moist towelettes in your pocket or purse for quick and convenient hand-wiping, suggests David N.F. Fairbanks, M.D., clinical professor of otolaryngology at George Washington University School of Medicine in Washington, D.C. If someone at home is already sick, cleaning surfaces will also help prevent germs from spreading.

Stay far from the sniffling crowd. December through February is flu season—not exactly the best time to mingle. After all, a single sneeze can propel virus-laden nose droplets about 12 feet. So it might be a good idea to stay away from cramped social settings, at least when a virus has been rampaging through your community.

Choke off stress. The effects of stress on your body are nothing to sneeze at. In one study researchers at Carnegie Mellon University in Pittsburgh asked 420 people about the stress in their lives. Then they exposed them to cold viruses. The more highly stressed a person was, the more likely he was to catch a cold.

Scientists suspect that stress releases hormones that suppress your immune system, making you more vulnerable to colds and other infections. But studies show that simple relaxation techniques like slow, deep breathing can help the immune system be more vigilant.

Stay true to your treadmill. In studies with couch-potato types, researchers at Appalachian State University in Boone, North Carolina, have found that several months of regular walking cuts in half the number of days with cold symptoms. And 80 percent of avid exercisers claim that regular training makes them less vulnerable to illness, compared with their former sedentary selves and their peers.

"Exercise has an activating effect on your body's immune, or surveillance, system," says lead researcher David C. Nieman, Dr.P.H., professor of health and exercise science at the university.

The key, says Dr. Nieman, is frequency. "In studies the biggest benefits accrue when you do an aerobic workout almost every day, at least five days a week, for 45 minutes to an hour at a time. If your symptoms are limited to the area from the neck up—like nasal stuffiness—going out for a walk might even help. But if your symptoms are below the neck, such as general muscle aches or chest congestion, or if you have a fever, it's best to lay off until you're up to par. Then gradually return to your normal routine," he says.

Stomp out the smokes. Cigarette smoke paralyzes the protective, hairlike cilia in your airways that help sweep viral mucus from your body. This is why smokers are far more likely to catch colds than nonsmokers.

Keep your house humid. "Mother Nature's way of preventing infections from taking hold is a moist mucous blanket that coats the nose and sinuses and sweeps viruses, dust particles, bacteria, and pollutants down the back of the throat," explains Dr. Fairbanks. "When your nose dries out, this blanket gets sluggish and slows way down, giving viruses a better chance to invade tissues."

It's not so much a problem for people who live in a part of the country that's dry year-round, since noses adapt and produce more mucus. But if you live in a region that requires heat for just one season, it's a good idea to humidify your home. Keep your humidifier squeaky clean. Empty leftover water, rinse, and refill with clean water daily. To deter the growth of bacteria, most humidifiers ideally should be washed weekly with 1 cup of bleach diluted in 1 gallon of water. Always check the manufacturer's cleaning instructions.

Strike Back at Colds and Flu

Even the best preventive measures won't insure that you'll never get another cold or flu. But if, despite your finest efforts, you still end up with a sore throat, the sniffles, and sneezes there are lots of after-the-fact remedies to soothe symptoms and speed you to recovery. Here's a sampling.

Suck on zinc. In a preliminary study from the Cleveland Clinic, 50 people who sucked on zinc lozenges every couple of hours had significantly shorter colds than people sucking on fake lozenges—4.4 days versus 7.6 days. They also suffered fewer days with runny noses, congestion, coughing, and sore throats.

"Right now, zinc looks better than anything else for treating the common cold," says Michael Macknin, M.D., study author and chairman of the department of general pediatrics at the clinic.

Two side effects occurred with the lozenges: About 20 percent of participants experienced nausea (though no one vomited), and up to 80 percent found the lozenges distasteful—sometimes intolerably so. Still, 90 percent of people completed the study.

The lozenges, called Cold-Eeze, are now available at many drugstores and some health food stores. Or write to the Quigley Corporation, P.O. Box 1349, Doylestown, PA 18901 for more information.

It's important to take zinc for only as long as cold symptoms last, says Dr. Macknin. Further studies are still needed to confirm these findings.

Take a plunge. Hot baths are among the best and simplest water treatments for a cold, according to Charles Thomas, Ph.D., a physical therapist at Desert Springs Therapy Center in Desert Hot Springs, California, and co-author of *Hydrotherapy: Simple Treatments for Common Ailments*. Here's what he recommends: Fill your tub with comfortably hot water (102° to 104°F; you can use a thermometer to check) and submerge as much of your body as possible. Soak for about 15 minutes. Towel off, jump into a prewarmed bed, and rest for at least 1 hour or longer (be sure to keep yourself warm, with your arms and legs well-covered). Dr. Thomas says to use this treatment one to three times every day until your symptoms subside.

Blaze a homeopathic trail. Oscillococcinum, Flu Solution, and other commercial homeopathic combination remedies containing duck liver and heart extract are excellent flu fighters, says Mitchell Fleisher, M.D., a family practice physician and homeopath in Colleen, Virginia. These remedies (available at health food stores) are particularly effective if taken in the first 4 to 12 hours after you start having symptoms. Follow the dosage on the label of the remedy you choose, he says. If it's going to work, you should feel relief with a single dose, he adds.

Hit influenza A with an antiviral. If your symptoms come on suddenly or include a fever, it probably means that you have a flu (which tends to start with a sore throat and meander its way into your nose and head). Call your local health bureau and find out what kind of flu is going around. If it's influenza A, call your doctor immediately. If you get a prescription antiviral like amantadine or rimantadine within the first 48 hours, you can stop the influenza A virus in its tracks.

Digestive Ailments

Reach for these age-old remedies to soothe heartburn, indigestion, irregularity, and other belly-wrenching ailments.

No matter how healthy you are, chances are that you've endured constipation, diarrhea, nausea, or another digestive problem that has sent you scrambling for a cure.

If the problem is stress-related—as it often is—it can be gently eased with natural medicine, says Michael Gershon, Ph.D., professor of anatomy and cell biology at the Columbia-Presbyterian Medical Center at Columbia University in New York City.

"People totally underestimate the impact of stress on the digestive system," states Kathleen Maier, a physician's assistant and herbalist who founded the Dreamtime Center for Herbal Studies in Flint Hill, Virginia, and former adviser on botanical medicine to the National Institutes of Health in Bethesda, Maryland. Alternative healers like Dr. Gershon and Maier, among others, say that stress-reducing natural therapies such as yoga and meditation have proved helpful to many people.

Grandma Was Right: Chew Your Food

Knowing how your digestive system is supposed to work is the first step in helping yourself prevent problems or heal them when things go wrong, says Maier. For instance, digestive problems can start when we don't take time out for simple rituals such as chewing our food properly and savoring what we eat, she explains. "So if your grandmother nagged you about chewing each bite of your food 100 times, she had good reasons," says Maier. Saliva contains specific enzymes that help break down complex carbohydrates. Without this enzymatic breakdown, food hasn't begun the proper digestive process.

But, of course, assiduous chewing isn't the only answer. Digestive problems have a wide range of possible causes. Many kinds of medications, including antibiotics and prescription steroids, can disturb intestinal peace. So can recreational drugs and alcohol. Any of these substances can wipe out beneficial bacteria, causing vague, unpleasant symptoms.

Natural approaches to digestive ills generally tackle problems from more than one angle, involving food therapy, vitamin and mineral therapy, herbal medicine, and some form of mind-body therapy, like yoga or meditation.

Constipation: Get Moving Naturally

You probably know the feeling only too well. You're bloated and you haven't, um, evacuated, for a couple of days. And now, you're getting pretty darn edgy. Constipation will do that to you.

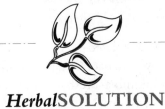

*Herbal*SOLUTION

These Teas Tame Indigestion

Indigestion is a catchall word for problems with digestive functions. Symptoms can include heartburn (a burning feeling felt near your breastbone), nausea, cramps, belching, and flatulence. Stress is probably a catalyst for indigestion, though scientists aren't exactly sure why. Eating too much or too fast is also commonly to blame.

One fast way to take the edge off indigestion is to use herbs, say natural healers. Here's what they recommend.

- Chamomile (*Chamomilla recutita*) or peppermint (*Mentha piperita*). "Chamomile and peppermint teas are wonderful for soothing tension-induced digestive troubles," says Andrew Weil, M.D., professor of herbalism and director of the Program of Integrative Medicine at the University of Arizona College of Medicine, near Tucson, and best-selling author of *Spontaneous Healing* and *Health and Healing*.

   "When you make the tea, be sure to keep the tea pot and your cup covered so that the vapor can't evaporate. A travel mug with

Estimates suggest that at least once in a while, 50 million Americans get that internal going-nowhere-fast feeling, while 18 million are often troubled by it. Fortunately, nature has ways to ease things along. Here are some of the best natural remedies for irregularity.

Shake, rattle, and roll. Exercise is an ideal way to jog your system into action. "The good muscle tone that results from a regular exercise program is important for optimal bowel function," says Maier. She recommends a brisk walk of a mile or two each day.

Fuel up on fiber. A high-fiber diet is the answer for constipation, says Julian Whitaker, M.D., founder of the Whitaker Wellness Center in Newport Beach, California. Most Americans eat only between 11 and 18 grams of fiber a day, he explains, but experts say that if you're constipated, you should shoot for more than 35 grams, the amount that you'd get from eating five servings of fresh fruits and vegetables as well as a heaping serva lid works well. The volatile oils in the vapor are what make the teas work," says Dr. Weil. To be sure that you're getting pure chamomile, he advises buying the herb from an established health food store or other reputable source.

- Marsh mallow (*Althaea officinalis*). Teas made from the soothing herb marsh mallow are excellent aids for your digestive system, says Kathleen Maier, a physician's assistant and herbalist who founded the Dreamtime Center for Herbal Studies in Flint Hill, Virginia, and former adviser on botanical medicine to the National Institutes of Health in Bethesda, Maryland. To make marsh mallow tea, use 1 tablespoon of dried herb to 1 cup of boiling water steeped for a minimum of 40 minutes. You can drink a cup of this tea once a day.
- Angelica root (*Angelica archangelica*). This is good for treating indigestion, mild stomach cramps, and lack of appetite, according to Commission E, the German group of scientists that makes recommendations on herbal safety and effectiveness. The suggested daily dose is a tea made with 2 to 3 teaspoons of dried herb per cup of boiling water, or up to 1 teaspoon of tincture.

ing of high-fiber cereal, such as oat or wheat bran, each day.

It's best to work fiber into your diet gradually. Suddenly increasing your fiber intake can cause gas, cramps, and diarrhea, says Adriane Fugh-Berman, M.D., former head of field investigations for the Office of Alternative Medicine at the National Institutes of Health.

Make water a priority. Constipation is often a sign that you're not drinking enough water. So along with regular exercise and more fiber, drinking eight or more 8-ounce glasses of water a day can help provide relief, according to Maier.

Let apple juice stir things up. Apple juice works wonders because it contains sorbitol, a natural sugar with laxative properties. So a glass a day may be just what you need to get things moving again, according to James Scala, Ph.D., nutritionist and author of *Eating Right for a Bad Gut.*

Diarrhea: Putting a Stop to the Going

There's nothing subtle about the symptoms of diarrhea. The cramps are sharp, and the urge to go is frequent. But if diagnosing diarrhea is easy, tracking down its cause may not be.

An episode of diarrhea is often caused simply by eating foods to which you're sensitive. Some people have lactose intolerance or gluten sensitivity, so they have problems eating dairy or wheat foods. A sudden increase in fiber intake or high-sugar foods can also cause problems, as can gas-producing vegetables such as brussels sprouts and cabbage. Viral or bacterial infections can also irritate the intestine, causing the runs.

You've ruled out those suspects? Sudden stress, even subtle distress, can loosen your bowels. So can antacids, caffeine, antibiotics, and beverages sweetened with sorbitol.

You might even get diarrhea from your kids—and not just because they delight in pushing your stress buttons. Mothers of tots in day care are 10 to 25 percent more likely to acquire the runs than are moms of stay-at-home children, according to one study. That's because it's easy for diarrhea-causing bacteria or viruses to spread among groups of yet-to-be-toilet-trained toddlers. Your kids pick up the germs and pass them to their caregivers—and to you.

With any luck, though, your particular blast of diarrhea won't last more than three days, especially if you try these natural remedies.

Roll some slippery elm. "Slippery elm is my favorite diarrhea remedy," says Susun S. Weed, an herbalist and teacher from Woodstock, New York, and author of the *Wise Woman* herbal series. She also speaks widely on the medicinal use of herbs at medical gatherings.

"Take a few spoonfuls of slippery elm bark powder, found at health food stores, and blend it with honey until you can roll the mixture into small balls. Dust the balls with additional slippery elm powder, store in a closed container, and use as needed, says Weed.

"I like to store them in little cough-drop tins," says Weed. "At the first sign of diarrhea, let a ball dissolve slowly in your mouth and repeat as necessary." Slippery elm works because it contains a nutritive mucilage, which soothes intestinal irritation, she says.

Dry up some blueberries. In Europe, dried blueberries are highly recommended as an effective cure for simple diarrhea, notes Varro E. Tyler, Ph.D, Sc.D., former professor of pharmacognosy at Purdue University in West Lafayette, Indiana, and author of *The New Honest Herbal* and *Herbs of Choice.* They contain pectin, a binding agent that helps dry up the problems. The antidiarrheal work is done largely by astringent tannins formed during the drying process, he adds.

In his book Dr. Tyler suggests chewing and swallowing 3 tablespoons of dried blueberries. Or, boil the crushed dried berries in water for about 10 minutes and drink the strained tea.

If you can't find dried blueberries in a gourmet or health food store, you can dry fresh berries in the sun or on a tray in a low-heat (150°F) oven overnight. Depending on the intensity of the sun and the temperature, drying time varies. Dry until no moisture oozes out when you squeeze a berry. But don't eat fresh blueberries for diarrhea, cautions Dr. Tyler. They may actually have a laxative effect.

Hemorrhoids: Try These Herbal Healers

If you've had hemorrhoids, you know only too well why they are so very hated. Not only do hemorrhoids cause pain that's often severe but they also bleed sometimes. And when you see bright red blood in your stool, you may think that you're in serious trouble.

Even when they are painful, you don't need to be alarmed. "Hemorrhoids are swollen veins found in the anal canal below the rectum," says Max M. Ali, M.D., in his book *Hemorrhoids: No Laughing Matter.* Describing them as "little balloons filled with blood," Dr. Ali says that hemorrhoids are caused by constipation, bad bowel habits, or pregnancy. In fact, hemorrhoids are almost an inevitable condition of pregnancy because the fetus exerts extraordinary pressure on the rectum.

If you have hemorrhoids, here's how to ease them naturally.

Bulk up. Eat plenty of vegetables and grains or use psyllium-based fiber supplements, say doctors. Fiber adds bulk, which contributes to larger, softer stools, and, as you could guess, soft, bulky stools are easier on your hemorrhoids than hard, dry ones.

Dab on some witch hazel. Distilled witch hazel extract is a natural astringent, and astringents help shrink swelling. "Put witch hazel on a plain cotton pad, or use cotton pads like Tucks that are presoaked in witch hazel. Apply to your hemorrhoids as often as needed to ease discomfort," suggests Maier.

Make an herbal sitz bath. Make two strong herbal infusions from dried comfrey leaves and dried calendula flowers. Both herbs are known for their healing, anti-inflammatory, and soothing properties, says Maier. Mix 1 tablespoon per cup of boiling water using ½ tablespoon calendula and ½ tablespoon comfrey, she recommends.

To make an infusion, pour hot water over the herbs and let them steep. In a 1-quart canning jar add 4 tablespoons of the blend to 4 cups boiling water; cover and steep for 30 minutes. Strain the herbs, then add the infusion to a bathtub half-full of warm water. Sit in the bath for at least 20 minutes, recommends Maier. Do this once a day, or twice a day if hemorrhoids are very painful.

Smooth on an herbal salve. Like witch hazel, horse-chestnut salve has astringent properties that soothe and shrink swollen hemor- rhoidal tissues, says Maier. It's available at health food stores.

Irritable-Bowel Syndrome: All Quiet below the Belt

More than 20 million Americans may suffer from irritable-bowel syndrome (IBS), doctors say, making it one of the most common digestive disorders.

"Irritable-bowel syndrome is a catchall word for all sorts of digestive problems," says Dr. Scala. Often, it's alternating constipation and diarrhea. Certain foods and stressful conditions can cause incredible abdominal pain, diarrhea, and even rectal bleeding. And the problem tends to be fre- quent or constant.

Because it has so many forms, IBS is known by a multitude of other names, such as spastic colitis, mucous colitis, spastic colon, or functional bowel disease. If you have true colitis, the lining of the bowel is inflamed, infected, or even ulcerated. There's none of these specific problems with IBS, even though the symptoms may resemble those of colitis.

The best ways to heal an irritable bowel are to modify your diet and your lifestyle. Here's what Dr. Scala recommends.

Dodge red meat. Stick to a vegetarian diet or at least avoid red meat, suggests Dr. Scala. Fish is fine. Or, have some skinless turkey or chicken breast. You can also have the meat from game animals such as rabbit and deer that were raised on grasses instead of corn, he adds.

Make those veggies well-done. Your cookbook may tell you to steam green, yellow, and orange vegetables till they're crisp-tender or al dente. But if you have IBS, Dr. Scala says, "Cook your vegetables till they're soft. You want to eliminate any sharp edges that can cause irritation." And, of course, completely raw vegetables are not advisable.

Go soft on hard foods. Be wary of chunky, sharp-edged foods, such as nuts. "Hard foods like nuts and seeds are more irritating than softer foods," says Dr. Scala.

If your love of hard foods makes eliminating them from your diet too difficult, then make sure that you chew them well, says Dr. Fugh-Berman.

Nausea and Vomiting: Fight the Urge to Purge

No matter what its cause—illness or tainted food, motion sickness or drinking too much—once the wave of nausea overtakes you, vomiting is almost sure to follow.

But sometimes vomiting doesn't follow, and you're stuck with the nausea—that queasy, not-quite-but-almost-dizzy feeling that starts in your stomach. When nausea lingers, you'll know exactly why cartoon characters who feel nauseated are colored green.

For very welcome relief from nausea, turn to the world of natural remedies.

Hone in on homeopathic helpers. "If you can match your symptoms to the correct remedy, using homeopathy at home can stem sudden, severe vomiting and nausea," says Michael Carlston, M.D., assistant clinical professor at the University of California, San Francisco, School of Medicine.

"In my experience some over-the-counter homeopathic medicines can relieve nausea and vomiting, especially if they contain the proper remedy for your specific symptoms," says Dr. Carlston. He recommends reading labels carefully to find out whether the remedy fits the symptoms that you're having.

For motion sickness that's more dizziness than nausea, Dr. Carlston suggests trying Cocculus, a homeopathic remedy derived from the Indian cockle. If the nausea outweighs the dizziness, use Tabacum, a remedy made from the tobacco plant. With both remedies, follow the label directions and look for potencies of 6C or 12C, suggests Dr. Carlston. The "C" indicates a homeopathic remedy's level of concentration.

Reach for ginger. Ginger is Chinese medicine's answer to Dramamine, the over-the-counter motion sickness medicine.

"It's a wonderful anti-nausea remedy," says Maier. "Whenever you feel queasy, grate a teaspoonful of fresh ginger into a hot cup of tea or eat some crystallized ginger candy." You can find this candy in gourmet or health food stores.

Nix nausea with a wristband. Acupressure, the ancient Chinese healing art, is the basis for a modern remedy that scientists say can control nausea and vomiting.

A simple wristband, called Sea-Band, presses a bead into a spot on the underside of your wrist, a spot associated with relief of nausea by those who practice the oriental arts of acupressure and acupuncture. The effectiveness of the wristband was supported by a German research team that found that women who wore the bands for 24 hours after minor gynecological surgery were able to reduce postsurgical nausea and vomiting by 50 percent. You can find Sea-Bands in health food stores and in some drugstores.

Fatigue

If you're feeling lethargic, take heart. We've uncovered some instant energizers that should help you power up when you're pooped.

There are days (though we find fewer of them as we get older) when our energy reserves seem limitless. We can go from task to complicated task all day and still have enough zip at night to mow the lawn, scrub the bathroom, and run a marathon. More often than not, however, we end our long days with about as much extra juice as a five-year-old car battery on a 10-degree day.

Here are some tips that can help you feel fully charged all day long.

Stoke your furnace each morning. Skipping breakfast isn't smart. "Research with students has shown that those who don't eat breakfast can't pay attention as well by 10:00 or 11:00 A.M.," says Jay Kenney, R.D., Ph.D., a nutrition research specialist at the Pritikin Longevity Center in Santa Monica, California. "The same is true for adults. We run out of steam."

Not all breakfasts are equal energy-wise. A high-sugar breakfast leaves you feeling mentally fatigued about an hour later. That's because it causes a spike in your blood sugar: First your blood sugar soars, then your system responds with insulin, which quashes both the sugar and your energy. The best breakfast to eat is oatmeal because it doesn't cause such spikes.

Have a tall, cold . . . water. Dehydration may trigger fatigue because it handicaps cells, says E. Wayne Askew, Ph.D., director of the division of foods and nutrition at the University of Utah in Salt Lake City. So stay ahead of dehydration by drinking 8 to 16 ounces of cold water as soon as you wake up, since your body is already facing a water deficit from the night.

Drink at least eight 8-ounce glasses of nonalcoholic, caffeine-free fluids each day, suggests William J. Evans, Ph.D., director of the Noll Physiological Research Center and professor of applied physiology and nutrition at Pennsylvania State University in University Park.

Don't pack it in. Just one high-fat, high-sugar meal can make you feel sluggish for hours afterward, Dr. Kenney says. A better approach is to eat a little bit of a healthy, high-fiber food like apples at least every 4 hours to help you stay alert.

Pick on a shrimp. When you're feeling lethargic and blue, order shrimp cocktail. Shrimp and other seafoods are high in the element selenium, which may lift your spirits. A study by the U.S. Department of Agriculture found that men who consumed 3½ times the daily recommended intake of selenium felt significantly more clear-headed and upbeat than men whose diets were low in the nutrient. You'll also find selenium in grains, poultry, and meats.

Find power in the simple things. You can get just as many, or even more, energy-packed carbohydrates from foods such as raisins, fig bars, and low-fat granola bars as you can from the average sports bar, says Nancy Clark, R.D., director of nutrition services at Sports Medicine Brookline in Massachusetts. As a bonus, you can save some money. The average granola bar costs about 30 cents, compared with the $1.00 or $2.00 performance bars.

Lay off the alcohol. Alcohol may relax you initially, but when your body metabolizes it hours later, some of the resulting compounds are

*Herbal*SOLUTION

Try the King of Zing

After years and years of contradictory and controversial study, evidence is finally emerging that ginseng, *Panax ginseng* (Asian) or *Panax quinquefolius* (American), can recharge the body, says Varro E. Tyler, Ph.D., Sc.D., former professor of pharmacognosy at Purdue University in West Lafayette, Indiana, and author of *The New Honest Herbal* and *Herbs of Choice*.

Two reliable investigations in the 1990s—one from Sweden involving 205 people and another from Mexico with 338 people—showed that ginseng, in combination with vitamins and minerals, resulted in improved quality of life. Other studies report improvements in memory and fatigue reduction, according to Dr. Tyler. And Commission E, the German panel entrusted with evaluating the safety and efficacy of herbal remedies, concluded that ginseng is a "tonic for invigoration and fortification in times of fatigue and debility, for declining capacity for work and concentration, and also during convalescence."

When buying ginseng capsules, look for products containing 4 percent ginsenoside (the active ingredient) extracted from Asian or American ginseng. Avoid imitation products made from Siberian, Brazilian, or Indian ginseng, Dr. Tyler urges. These products are less effective than those made from Asian or American forms of the herb. The recommended dose of a typical product containing 4 percent ginsenosides is two 100-milligram capsules daily, he says.

stimulants. A drink after dinner may help you fall asleep sooner, but 2 to 3 hours later, you'll wake up. And that never makes for a good night's sleep.

Plus, alcohol dehydrates you, and dehydration can make you feel tired. "If you drink a lot of alcohol one day, it may take you another entire day to drink enough fluids to make up for it," Dr. Evans says.

Put a lid on caffeine. Coffee, tea, and other products containing caffeine can disturb sleep and ultimately make you feel fatigued. "Some people can't sleep if they eat just a little piece of chocolate cake after dinner. Others can take much more. You have to read labels, know your limits, and respect them," says Peter Hauri, Ph.D., director of the Mayo Clinic's insomnia program in Rochester, Minnesota.

See the light. A lack of natural light, particularly in the winter months, can make some people feel sad and tired, says Kathryn A. Lee, R.N., Ph.D., professor of family health care nursing at the University of California, San Francisco. She suggests taking a walk in the morning or mid-afternoon. "Even a short walk on a cloudy day can give you some of the light that you need," she says.

Sleep an extra hour. This means going to bed an hour earlier. Sleep expert Mary A. Carskadon, Ph.D., professor of psychiatry at Brown University in Providence, Rhode Island, monitored 66 students before and after extending their usual sleeping time an hour or two each night. The result was that students felt much more alert and energetic after sleeping longer.

Break things up. Rather than slog through a tedious task until it is finished and you collapse, take short breaks. Research suggests that breaks actually speed up work, making you more productive and less fatigued, according to Harold H. Bloomfield, M.D., and Robert K. Cooper, Ph.D., authors of *The Power of 5*.

Switch headache remedies. Taking ibuprofen for a headache or muscle soreness can make you sleepy since nonsteroidal anti-inflammatory drugs (NSAIDs) can be sedating for some people. If NSAIDs affect you this way, try substituting acetaminophen or aspirin.

Get on your feet. Instead of depleting your resources, exercise increases your energy. Just as it makes your heart work better, exercise helps your brain function more efficiently. It also has an antidepressive effect, possibly because it boosts levels of neurotransmitters like endorphins.

While almost any exercise can help fight fatigue, the best is aerobic exercise. It doesn't matter if you ride a bike or walk briskly around the block. Whatever aerobic activity you choose, doing it for a minimum of 20 minutes two or three times a week will help improve circulation, muscle tone, and even your outlook, experts say.

Headaches and Migraines

*Whether caused by stress, tension, noise, light, or eating
the wrong foods, headaches have one thing in common—
they hurt. But an amazing number of nondrug
approaches can bring relief.*

It throbs, it bangs, it squeezes. It's a pain like no other, and few of us have been fortunate enough to escape it. In fact, more than 90 percent of Americans have at least one headache in their lifetime. Nearly 60 percent of men and more than 75 percent of women probably have had at least one headache in the past month.

If you're one of the them, you don't want to hear about how you should have slept more, had less to drink, or left your computer screen a few hours ago. You want to know how to stop the pain. Here's your checklist.

Change the bulb. The constant, barely perceptible flickering of fluorescent light tubes can bring on a blinding headache. Kill the overhead light and bring in a few lamps with regular incandescent bulbs, suggests Lawrence Robbins, M.D., author of *Headache Help.*

Take a mental vacation. Guided imagery is a very effective way to rid yourself of headaches, says Dennis Gersten, M.D., a psychiatrist in San Diego and publisher of *Atlantis: The Imagery Newsletter.* To try it, sit or lie in a comfortable position and close your eyes. Imagine that you are lying on a beach with the sun comfortably warming you. The waves gently pour over you. Each time the waves roll back out to sea, they pull more and more tension out of your body.

After you're relaxed, Dr. Gersten suggests trying this imagery: Focus your attention on your headache. Imagine that the pain has a certain size, shape, and color. What does it feel like? Is it smooth or rough? Does it stay in one place in your head or does it move around? Allow the headache to turn to liquid. Allow the pain to roll down into your neck, then down into one shoulder, into your hand, and finally, your fingertips. Then allow the liquid to pour out of your fingertips and watch it as it flows out into the room or the space that you are in.

Have a head cold. Wrap a bag of crushed ice in a towel and hold it to the area of your head that hurts. This technique works best for headaches that are characterized by dull throbs. The cold reduces the inflammation of the blood vessels that causes pain.

Have some caffeine. Try having a cup of coffee, advises Fred Sheftell, M.D., co-founder and co-director of the New England Center for Headache in Stamford, Connecticut. He says that caffeine constricts blood vessels and is an ingredient in many pain relievers. In fact, studies show that having a cup of coffee or tea can boost the pain-relieving powers of aspirin and other such products by about one-third.

Skim the fat. Research suggests that if you cut back on fat, you may cut back on headaches, too. When 54 people with regular migraines spent a month flushing most of the fat out of their diets, their headaches were less frequent, less intense, and shorter in duration, and they needed fewer medications, according to a report published in the medical journal *Headache.*

Researchers think that fat may mess with your head through a chain reaction involving blood factors called platelets. Fat encourages platelets to congregate, and in the process, the platelets damage each other, which results in release of the brain chemical serotonin into the blood. This temporary high level of serotonin is then quickly metabolized and excreted,

Unplug Phony Headaches

If your usually cool head is suddenly hot with a headache, don't be so quick to blame it on the loud voice in the next office. It could be what you're using to try to block the noise out.

Doctors were at first puzzled by one 37-year-old woman's sudden, throbbing headache that spread to her neck, shoulders, and throat . . . until they learned that she had just spend two 8-hour days wearing headphones with hard plastic earpieces. Ann K. Skelton, M.D., explained in the *New England Journal of Medicine* that the pain was probably from earpieces that were pressing on the glossopharyngeal nerve (a portion of which lies in the ear). Pain disappeared when the woman stopped using the headset. This pressure headache is probably pretty rare, says Dr. Skelton. But the point is that if you're getting a migraine and you're not the headache-getting sort, don't assume that it's the start of a downward trend. Maybe all you need to do is disconnect—or change—the 'phones.

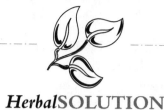

*Herbal*SOLUTION

Leaf Your Pain Behind

No single natural therapy—or pharmaceutical, for that matter—works for every type of headache, experts say. There are, however, several herbs that can help relieve the different types.

- Feverfew (*Tanacetum parthenium*). Eating a single leaf of the herb feverfew every day may help keep migraines and chronic headaches at bay, says Ethan Russo, M.D., neurologist at the Western Montana Clinic in Missoula, academic adjunct professor in the department of pharmacy at the University of Montana in Missoula, and clinical assistant professor in the department of medicine at the University of Washington School of Medicine in Seattle. "It's unknown how it works, but it's an anti-inflammatory and painkiller."

    Although you can buy feverfew capsules in health food stores, Dr. Russo says that you can't be sure of their quality. "I usually recommend growing a plant of your own," he notes. "You can get seed anywhere that you can get herbs. Your best bet is to try to find a local supplier of fresh herbs, or look through seed catalogs. It's not a hard plant to grow."

    One caveat: Pregnant women should not take feverfew because of a remote possibility that it might trigger miscarriage,

leaving a low level of serotonin in the blood. With a stingy amount of serotonin, blood vessels are known to widen and roll out the red carpet to a migraine, says study leader Zuzana Bic, M.D., Dr.P.H., of the preventive care program at Loma Linda University School of Public Health in California.

Dr. Bic recommends a diet that is no more than 10 percent of calories from fat. In the study researchers found success with cutbacks to an ultralow 20 grams of fat (or about 10 percent of calories from fat) in people who had previously been eating 80 to 120 grams of fat per day. The key, Dr. Bic believes, isn't to replace fatty foods with nonfat processed options. Instead, reach for more fruits, vegetables, legumes, and grains.

says James A. Duke, Ph.D., a retired U.S. Department of Agriculture botanist and author of *The Green Pharmacy*. And women who are nursing should not use it because of the possibility of passing the herb to infants through milk. Finally, long-term users often report a mild tranquilizing or sedative effect, which may be welcome or unwelcome, depending on your temperament.

- Willow bark (*Salix*, various species). Commission E, the group of experts that advises the German government about herbs, endorses willow bark as an effective pain reliever for headache and anything else treated by willow's pharmaceutical derivative, aspirin.

  When herbalists talk about willow bark as herbal aspirin, they usually mention the white willow (*Salix alba*). But this species is rather low in salicin, the aspirin-like chemical in the bark that relieves pain. If you want more headache relief per cup of tea, there are other willow species that are more potent, such as *S. daphnoides*, *S. fragilis*, or *S. purpurea*. Commission E recommends getting 60 to 120 milligrams of salicin to treat a headache, which works out to 1 teaspoon of the high-salicin barks, or 1 to 1½ teaspoons of white willow.

- Evening primrose (*Oenothera biennis*) is one of the best sources of the pain-relieving compound phenylalanine, Dr. Duke says. For those with chronic headaches, nutritionists may recommend a daily dose of 6 to 8 capsules of evening primrose oil.

Take a breather. Sometimes, stopping everything that you're doing and simply breathing deeply can work wonders for tension headaches, says Joseph P. Primavera III, Ph.D., psychologist and co-director of the Comprehensive Headache Center at Germantown Hospital and Medical Center in Philadelphia. "Stop doing whatever you were doing that was stressful," he suggests. Take slow, deep, rhythmic breaths. Breathing this way alters your carbon dioxide level and sends a message to your brain to slow your heartbeat and promote the relaxation response."

A quick way to take a breather is by slowly taking a deep inhalation through your mouth, filling up your lungs, and then taking a full respiration through your nose and breathing out nice and slow, Dr. Primavera says.

Seek homeopathic relief. In their book, *The Complete Guide to Homeopathy,* Andrew Lockie, M.D., and Nicola Geddes, M.D., suggest the following homeopathic remedies for migraines, depending on your symptoms. Homeopathic remedies are available at most health food stores.

If the migraine is worse on the left side, with severe nausea and vomiting and pain that extends to the face, mouth, or teeth, the remedy is taking 6C of ipecac every 15 minutes for up to 10 doses. (Homeopathic remedies are available in different potencies, or concentrations, expressed by a number and commonly followed by the letter "C.")

If it's a blinding, throbbing migraine that begins with numbness and tingling in the lips and tongue and the pain is severe and pulsating, the remedy is taking 6C of nux vomica every hour for up to six doses.

If it's a migraine that settles over the right eye, usually starting in the morning at the back of the head and spreading up to the forehead, the remedy is sanguinaria, which should be taken at the first sign of an attack, in a dosage of 6C every 15 minutes for up to 10 doses.

Note: If you don't improve within the time period noted on the remedy package, or if you experience chronic migraines, see a physician. If a headache follows a head injury, or if it's severe and associated with a fever or lasts more than a few days, seek immediate medical assistance.

Turn to magnesium. See your doctor about this one. A study at the New York Headache Center in New York City found that a shot of magnesium can relieve severe migraine or cluster headaches within 15 minutes. The shots worked only for people who had low magnesium levels, but there's a 50-50 chance that you're one of them, says Alexander Mauskop, M.D., who directed the study. Oral supplements don't have the same effect, but daily doses may prevent migraines. Dr. Mauskop recommends 500 milligrams of chelated (check the label) magnesium, divided into two or three doses through the day.

Pepper up. Rubbing capsaicin (the stuff that makes red pepper hot) on your nose can relieve cluster headaches. Ask your doctor for a capsaicin preparation. It helped 75 percent of people in one study. But avoid getting it in your eyes, because it may cause irritation.

Rinse your nose out. Irrigating your sinuses is a good solution for sinus headaches, says Thomas M. Kidder, M.D., associate professor of otolaryngology and human communication at the Medical College of Wisconsin in Milwaukee. To unclog nasal passages, make a saline solution from 1 level teaspoon of table salt and 13 ounces of warm water, and then sniff it into your nose through cupped hands. Or take a bulb syringe and squirt it into your nose. "If you squirt it into the congested nostril and lean forward, the saline will drain out the other nostril. It cleans out the nose and the thick secretions that you get there," Dr. Kidder says.

Give the pain a rub. Getting a head massage can be a soothing experience, says Paul Petit, D.C., a certified chiropractic sports physician, aromatherapist, and naturopath in Poway, California. It's not always easy to drop everything and head for a massage therapist every time you have a headache. But you can deeply massage the back of your head where the cranium starts and the vertebrae stop, and the temples on either side of your eyes, which are definite pressure points during headaches. "I'd say that you need a deep massage of the area for 10 to 20 minutes," Dr. Petit says. "Those points act as an accessory pump to your brain, so this helps get your blood pumping, relaxing constricted blood vessels."

Heart Disease

Even if your family has a history of heart disease, there are many things that you can do to improve the odds in your favor. The key is to know, monitor, and change the risk factors that you can control.

Imagine cutting your risk of heart disease to zero. Impossible? Not for most of us. With reams of data collected over decades of research, we have a pretty darn good idea why some people get heart disease and some don't. It all boils down to risk factors. And, as it turns out, almost all of these risk factors are within your control . . . and the one that isn't (family history) usually can be minimized by controlling the others.

Who says? One of America's foremost heart doctors, William P. Castelli, M.D. As director of the famed Framingham Heart Study in Massachusetts, the largest, longest research project designed to assess risk factors for coronary artery disease, Dr. Castelli has spent the past 30 years poring over the findings. And by practicing what he's learned, he knows

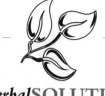

*Herbal*SOLUTION

Natural Heart Menders Abound

Garlic, onion, ginger, and red pepper help prevent and treat heart attack by reducing blood pressure. Garlic and onions also cut cholesterol and discourage the blood from forming internal clots, according to James A. Duke, Ph.D., a retired U.S. Department of Agriculture botanist and author of *The Green Pharmacy*. If you know much about herbs, that information probably isn't news to you. But you may not know that many other herbs can help prevent and treat heart disease as well. Here are a couple of heart-strengthening herbs suggested by Dr. Duke.

- Pigweed (*Amaranthus*, various species) and other plants containing calcium. Pigweed leaves are one of our best plant sources of calcium (about 5.3 percent on a dry-weight basis). Studies suggest that calcium adds mineral density to bone, which can help prevent osteoporosis. But there's more: The mineral also significantly reduces heart attack risk.

  Other high-calcium plants include lamb's quarter, stinging nettle, broad beans, watercress, licorice, marjoram, savory, red clover shoots, and thyme.

  In addition to calcium, pigweed is high in fiber. A six-year Harvard study of more than 40,000 men showed that compared with those who consumed the least fiber, those who ate the most had

firsthand the remarkable power that each of us wields against this killer disease. At age 64, he's still holding heart disease at bay, unlike every other male member of his family, who started showing signs in their forties.

The secret? "Know, monitor, and change controllable risk factors," says Dr. Castelli, now medical director of the Framingham Cardiovascular Institute. "If all Americans did this, heart disease would be eradicated, just as polio was," he says.

Here's what to do to ensure a disease-free future for your heart.

- Don't smoke. You know why.
- Walk 2 miles a day (or the equivalent in another form of exercise).

just one-third the risk of heart attack.

You can add pigweed to salads, mixed vegetable dishes, and minestrone.

• Willow bark (*Salix*, various species) contains salicin—the herbal precursor of aspirin. A great deal of research shows that low-dose aspirin—one-half to one standard tablet a day—can reduce heart attack risk substantially by preventing the internal blood clots that trigger it.

The body converts aspirin into salicylic acid. The body also converts the salicin in willow bark into salicylic acid. So if pharmaceutical aspirin helps prevent heart attack, herbal aspirin should, too. If you're allergic to aspirin, though, you probably shouldn't take herbal aspirin, either.

Typically, people use white willow bark (*S. alba*), but several other species are richer in salicin, including crack willow (*S. fragilis*) and purple osier (*S. purpurea*). But if white willow is the only kind that you can find at your health food store or herb shop, that's okay.

About ½ teaspoon (1 gram) of white willow bark contains approximately 100,000 parts per million of salicin, or about 100 milligrams. After conversion into salicylic acid, that should be about enough to have aspirin's heart-protective effect.

Dr. Duke suggests brewing a tea with a teaspoon or so of bark to a cup of boiling water. Steep for 15 minutes and strain. Drink a cup a day, or one every other day.

People who exercise regularly have a death rate from all causes, including heart disease, just one-quarter that of nonexercisers. If you haven't exercised at all in the past year, however, begin slowly and with your doctor's okay. If you've had a heart attack, you should make sure that you are monitored by your doctor.

• Decrease calories to maintain a healthy body weight. The Framingham Cardiovascular Institute starts all patients on a 2,000-calorie diet. This makes it easier to use the new nutrition-facts labels (all values are based on 2,000 calories).

(continued on page 174)

Determining Your Heart-Healthy Weight

Body mass index (BMI) is a simple formula that compares your height with your weight. Many doctors consider it a more accurate measure of your risk of heart disease and other ailments than other height/weight charts issued by Metropolitan Life Insurance Company or other authorities, such as the U.S. Department of Agriculture and the Department of Health and Human Services.

To calculate your BMI, divide your weight (in pounds) by your height (in inches) squared. If you're 130 pounds and 5 feet 3 inches tall, for example, that's 130 divided by 3,969 (63 × 63), which is 0.032. Multiply the number you get by 705 (0.032 × 705 = 23). The number that you get is your BMI. Or you can use the table below, which does all of the mathematics for you. Most likely, your BMI will fall somewhere between 19 and 32.

Several large-scale medical studies involving thousands of people have suggested that 21 to 22 is the optimal BMI. At this level there are

Height	Weight (lb.)						
4'10"	91	96	100	105	110	115	119
4'11"	94	99	104	109	114	119	124
5'0"	97	102	107	112	118	123	128
5'1"	100	106	111	116	122	127	132
5'2"	104	109	115	120	126	131	136
5'3"	107	113	118	124	130	135	141
5'4"	110	116	122	128	134	140	145
5'5"	114	120	126	132	138	144	150
5'6"	118	124	130	136	142	148	155
5'7"	121	127	134	140	146	153	159
5'8"	125	131	138	144	151	158	164
5'9"	128	135	142	149	155	162	169
5'10"	132	139	146	153	160	167	174
5'11"	136	143	150	157	165	172	179
6'0"	140	147	154	162	169	177	184
BMI	19	20	21	22	23	24	25

no weight-related health risks, according to William P. Castelli, M.D., medical director of the Framingham Cardiovascular Institute in Framingham, Massachusetts and director of the famed Framingham Heart Study. In a long-term study of 115,886 healthy women ages 30 to 55, researchers at Harvard and Brigham Women's hospital in Boston concluded that there was no elevated risk of heart disease among women whose BMIs were under 21. In comparison, the risk was 30 percent higher among women whose BMI was 21 to 25, 80 percent higher for a BMI of 25 to 29, and 230 percent higher for a BMI greater than 29.

So for your target weight, shoot for a BMI of no more than 21 or 22, Dr. Castelli recommends.

To find your BMI, locate your height in the left column. (If you've lost inches over the years, use your peak adult height.) Move across the chart to the right until you find your approximate weight. Then follow that column down to the corresponding BMI number at the bottom of the chart.

124	129	134	138	143	148	153
128	133	138	143	148	153	158
133	138	143	148	153	158	163
137	143	148	153	158	164	169
142	147	153	158	164	169	174
146	152	158	163	169	175	180
151	157	163	169	174	180	186
156	162	168	174	180	186	192
161	167	173	179	186	192	198
166	172	178	185	191	197	204
171	177	184	190	197	203	210
176	182	189	196	203	209	216
181	188	195	202	207	215	222
186	193	200	208	215	222	229
191	199	206	213	221	228	235
26	**27**	**28**	**29**	**30**	**31**	**32**

- Decrease overall dietary fat to no more than 55 grams daily (or no more than 25 percent of calories), based on a 2,000-calorie diet. Defatting your diet not only helps blood fat levels but it helps you shed pounds, too. That's because fat is the most concentrated source of calories. To limit total fat steer clear of bakery goodies, snack foods (such as chips and packaged cookies), and deep-fried foods (especially fast foods).

- Decrease saturated fat to no more than 20 grams daily (10 grams if you've suffered a heart attack). "But these are absolute maximums," says Dr. Castelli. "Anything less is better." Saturated fats in the diet are the number one contributor to bad blood fats. To limit

Being Frisky Is Not So Risky

If you've had a heart attack, research suggests "don't worry, be frisky." Scientists have found that sexual activity poses no danger to your heart.

Researchers at Harvard Medical School questioned 858 heart attack patients to see how many had sex in the 2 hours before their heart attacks—the window of time that's considered the hazard period for heart attack triggers. They then looked at the chance that sex was actually the cause of a heart attack (just because someone had a heart attack after sex doesn't mean that the heart attack was caused by sex).

While the risk was twice as high for those with heart disease, it's not cause for alarm: That doubling of risk actually represented a two-in-a-million risk of heart attack versus a one-in-a-million chance. If you want to whittle down that risk even further, the best thing to do is exercise.

Those with heart disease who exercised three or more times a week had only a tiny bit higher risk (1.2 times) than their peers who didn't have heart disease. People with heart disease who didn't exercise at all, however, had three times the risk of couch potatoes who didn't have heart disease. That means that getting off the couch to exercise three times a week could cut your already low risk by two-thirds.

The findings could have a major positive impact on those afraid to enjoy sex, says Robert F. DeBusk, M.D., director of the Cardiac Rehabilitation Program at Stanford University School of Medicine. "After all," he says, "people are interested not only in the years in their lives, but also in the liveliness of their years."

saturated fats avoid butter and dairy products like whole and 2% milk, high-fat cheese, and high-fat ice cream. Limit meat servings to 3 to 4 ounces daily. Choose only select-grade meats, trim all visible fat, and prepare by broiling or grilling without added fat. Limit low-fat cheese to 1 or 2 ounces daily; and when you do include it, decrease meat by the same number of ounces that you increased cheese.

- Decrease dietary cholesterol to no more than 300 milligrams daily (200 milligrams if you've had a heart attack). By restricting saturated fat you usually automatically restrict cholesterol—with one major exception: egg yolks. Most people who have had a heart attack, and even those who haven't had them, should use egg whites only or cholesterol-free egg substitutes. Bakery products can also be high in cholesterol, so be sure to restrict those as well. (They're also generally high in fat and refined carbohydrates.)

- Decrease sodium intake. Although not everyone is sensitive to salt's blood pressure–raising ability, there is no way to predict who is. That's why Dr. Castelli recommends that everyone cut sodium intake from the average American intake of 10,000 milligrams to just 1,250 milligrams per day. (That translates to 2,500 milligrams of salt per day.) The easiest way? "Cut down on processed, canned, and convenience foods and don't use salt in cooking," says Dr. Castelli. It's a good idea to keep the saltshaker off the table, too.

- If you're a woman at or near menopause, consider hormone-replacement therapy (HRT). Research has shown that women who take HRT have half the heart attack rate of women who don't take it. Dr. Castelli suggests that all women, especially those with a strong family history combined with elevated risk factors, consider taking postmenopausal estrogen.

- Find an outlet for your stress. Stress negatively impacts many body systems and can have a measurable impact on blood pressure. Dr. Castelli advises his patients to identify a stress-reduction strategy that works well for them—meditation, deep breathing, regular exercise, and massage, to name just a few—and to stick with it.

High Blood Pressure

Only one in four Americans with high blood pressure (hypertension) receives proper treatment, according to some health care experts. But this "silent killer" can be tamed if you and your doctor avoid these common mistakes.

The news slipped in quietly, like a kid tiptoeing in the back door with a bad report card. Maybe that's because the news was a don't-tell-Mom kind of grade. Members of the American College of Cardiology, the American College of Preventive Medicine, and six other health care groups had taken a look at the treatment of high blood pressure in this country and found it wanting. They gave it a C minus. Go to the back of the class.

That wasn't the only dunce cap issued. The National Heart, Lung, and Blood Institute also released a statement saying that 50 percent of the high blood pressure in the United States is either undetected or inadequately treated.

But "the statistics are even a little worse," says Harry Gavras, M.D., vice-chairman of the American Heart Association's Council for High Blood Pressure Research and chief of the hypertension and atherosclerosis section of Boston University Medical Center. Thirty-five percent of people with high blood pressure don't even know that they have the problem, and 27 percent are inadequately treated. Only 25 percent are adequately or well-treated.

That's a shame, because high blood pressure is a risk factor for heart attack, stroke, and congestive heart failure. And 50 million of us have it. High blood pressure makes us five times more prone to strokes, three times more likely to have heart attacks, and two to three times more likely to suffer congestive heart failure. But guess what? It's reversible.

It's also sneaky and sly, the "silent killer." So it's understandable that one-third of the folks who have it don't know. A stubbed toe produces more pain. With high blood pressure blood rushes through your vessels like a soundless speedboat. You don't feel it, but over time the force of that ride damages the blood vessels' surfaces. Fatty debris sticks easily to rough walls then. The vessels narrow. Clots can form and break loose, causing a heart attack or stroke. Even if that doesn't happen, the heart labors and

Can Shut-Eye Shut Off Hypertension?

After last night's late ending, you think that you might need Hercules to pry you out of bed. But by the time the sun edges into view, your blood pressure may have already risen. Maybe even to a peak.

Preliminary research suggests that staying awake during your usual sleeping hours—trying to finish that quilt for your niece or even just being out late—may create a surge of extra pressure in your blood vessels.

Blood pressure tends to go down when we sleep and gets fired up again at waking time. But when 18 healthy people had a hard day's night—they went to bed $3\frac{1}{2}$ hours later than usual but stuck to their typical reveille—their blood pressure readings, although still within a normal range, were significantly higher in the morning than they were after a standard 8-hour night of sleep. Their heart rates were higher after a sleep-deprived night, too.

No one knows for sure whether these morning-after power surges mean persistent high blood pressure later. Nor is it clear that these spikes are a cause of the large number of heart attacks that occur in the morning.

But the pressure jump in the study is a fairly clear sign that burning the midnight oil (or party lights) stresses out your system, says Jerome Markovitz, M.D., a blood pressure researcher at the University of Alabama in Birmingham.

Experts suspect that sleep deprivation might increase adrenaline and therefore drive up blood pressure and especially heart rate. That could be because the body has to work overtime just trying to keep itself awake, says sleep expert Michael Bonnet, Ph.D., professor of neurology at Wright State University and director of the sleep lab at the Veterans Administration Hospital, both in Dayton, Ohio.

Such pressure spikes may have immediate implications if you prefer early-morning doctor visits. Pressure measured after a bad night may go on record as higher than usual. If you're monitoring your own blood pressure and on some mornings readings are sky-high, note whether you slept well the night before.

If it seems that you're jotting down difficulty sleeping every night, try clearing your schedule. See if someone else can do the laundry for a change. As Thoreau said, "Simplify, simplify, simplify." It may take a lot of the pressure off.

strains, weakening and enlarging.

For all the drama, it's mute theater. That's why you should get your pressure checked once a year. You need a stethoscope to hear it. Once heard, though, what explains the high incidence of below-par medical treatment? We asked five top blood pressure specialists and found out the five biggest mistakes that doctors make in high blood pressure treatment—and what you can do to prevent them.

#1: Doctors Rely on Too Few Measures

Here's what happens. "Patients get one high reading. Their doctors put them on medication. They come back and they're fine; the doctors say that the medication has done the trick. But in many cases, even without medication, the patients' pressures would have been fine," says Thomas G.

How to Choose a Monitor

Sure, stethoscopes were fun to play with when you were a kid. But they're not the easiest tools to maneuver when you're taking your own blood pressure. There are some blood pressure monitors that have addressed the ease of taking measurements, though, says Thomas G. Pickering, M.D., professor of medicine at the hypertension center at New York Hospital–Cornell Medical Center in New York City and author of *Good News about High Blood Pressure.*

One home blood pressure unit that Dr. Pickering likes incorporates the stethoscope on the blood pressure cuff. "It's reliable but still requires a certain degree of skill and hearing ability. So not everybody can use one," he says. Most people find electronic home units the easiest systems to manage. They read blood pressure via sensors and print out the reading.

Avoid the units that measure pressure from your finger or wrist. They're not reliable, says Dr. Pickering. And home monitors should be taken to a doctor's office to make sure that they're accurate, he says.

No matter which kind of monitor you purchase, test-drive the new machine alongside your doctor's to make sure that they're in sync. Then take it in once a year for an accuracy checkup. (The manual models aren't as touchy.)

Pickering, M.D., professor of medicine at the hypertension center at New York Hospital–Cornell Medical Center in New York City and author of *Good News about High Blood Pressure.*

That's because a blood pressure reading is just one brief snapshot in time. One reading may not at all represent what's going on most days. Government guidelines for treatment suggest multiple readings during each doctor's visit.

"Even then, our research has shown that for some people, doctors' readings are often the least representative of their overall levels of blood pressure," says Dr. Pickering. The reason is that about one in five people with high blood pressure suffers from "white-coat hypertension." Doctors' offices make them nervous. Their blood pressures spike. But they don't usually need to be medicated.

One way to get around that is to ask the doctor's nurse or technician to take your blood pressure. Another is to take your own blood pressure. "There's a big movement for home monitoring," says Dr. Pickering. You can buy manual or electronic home units that provide fairly reliable readings.

With a home monitor you can average out various readings taken during the course of a day. Your measurements may very well be different in the morning and evening, at work and after exercise. But you'll be able to get the total picture, especially if you track pressure for a few weeks and average out all the different readings.

#2: Doctors Don't Spend Enough Time Treating It

Too often, high blood pressure gets short shrift in doctors' offices. And there are two big reasons for this. "Part of the problem is that even though hypertension is extremely common, it's not generally recognized as a medical specialty. There are no board examinations to qualify as a specialist. And for most physicians it's not their prime interest. So hypertension frequently doesn't get the professional scrutiny that it needs. It's treated mostly by family practitioners, internists, nephrologists, and cardiologists," says Dr. Pickering.

The other part of the problem is the sheer amount of time that hypertension demands. "You have to give patients tender loving care. But it's hard to do on a 15-minute schedule. If you don't, though, you're doomed to failure," says Ray W. Gifford, Jr., M.D., professor of internal medicine at

Ohio State University College of Medicine in Columbus and consulting physician in the department of nephrology and hypertension at the Cleveland Clinic Foundation. "One of the most common mistakes is that doctors don't spend enough time up front convincing patients that the way to reduce their risks of stroke and heart attack is to lower their blood pressures. Then the doctors need to talk to their patients and make lifestyle changes tempting, because people tend to resist them. They have to make sure that patients know that those changes are almost sure to bring their blood pressure down, so they may not need medication.

"You can't tell patients to start a low-salt diet and an exercise program and come back in six months," Dr. Gifford says. "They need to come in three times during those six months to reinforce lifestyle modifications. They need a physician who spends the time to keep evaluating them once they're on a program."

But how do you find a dedicated doctor if you can't look him up in the Yellow Pages under "Hypertension Specialist, Long Hours"?

Dr. Pickering has formed the Hypertension Network, which makes use of the Internet to provide people with up-to-date information about hypertension, including question-and-answer forums. It can also provide a list of physicians who have a special interest in treating hypertension. The Web site address is http://www.bloodpressure.com. Or write to the Hypertension Network at P.O. Box 302, Wingdale, NY 12594.

If you don't want to look for a new physician because you already have a longtime family doctor you like, make an appointment for a heart-to-heart talk with him. Go prepared: Write down your questions and refer to them. If you've read up on the subject and made notes for discussion, bring them in, too. Tell your doctor your concerns about your blood pressure and its treatment. Let him know that you're willing to take an active role in managing your condition by recording your blood pressure and by making appropriate lifestyle changes.

#3: Doctors Hold Off Treatment

"This is a common problem—physicians often don't initiate therapy in patients with mild hypertension. They wait until the hypertension is worse. But this waiting game is considered a major public-health concern by all the experts in this area," says William B. White, M.D., chief of

*Herbal*SOLUTION

Breathtaking Herbs Ease High Blood Pressure

There are any number of herbs that can help control blood pressure, says James A. Duke, Ph.D., a retired U.S. Department of Agriculture botanist and author of *The Green Pharmacy*. Here are a couple of the better-known ones.

- Garlic (*Allium sativum*). This wonder herb not only helps normalize blood pressure but it also reduces cholesterol, Dr. Duke says. In a scientifically rigorous study done in 1993, people with high blood pressure were given about one clove of garlic a day for 12 weeks. Afterward, they exhibited significantly lower diastolic blood pressure and cholesterol levels. (Diastolic readings measure the amount of pressure produced by your heart between beats.)

  "We now know that garlic can reduce hypertension, even in quantities as small as ½ ounce per week," says Varro E. Tyler, Ph.D., Sc.D., former professor of pharmacognosy at Purdue University in West Lafayette, Indiana, and author of *The New Honest Herbal* and *Herbs of Choice*. One-half ounce per week works out to about one clove a day. If you cook with garlic and use it in your salads, getting that much should be a snap. If you haven't yet developed a taste for it, you can take garlic in capsule form, available over the counter at many drugstores, Dr. Duke says.

- Hawthorn (*Crataegus oxyacantha*) extract. This can widen (dilate) blood vessels, especially the coronary arteries, according to a report published in the Lawrence Review of Natural Products. Hawthorn has been used as a heart tonic for centuries, Dr. Duke says.

  If you'd like to try this powerful heart medicine, discuss it with your doctor. You can try a tea made with 1 teaspoon of dried herb per 1 cup of boiled water. Drink up to 2 cups a day, Dr. Duke suggests.

the section of hypertension at the University of Connecticut Health Center in Farmington. The fact is, even mild hypertension increases your risk of stroke and heart attack. Stage one (mild) hypertension means that your systolic reading (the top figure, which measures how hard your heart has to pump) is between 140 and 159 and your diastolic pressure (which measures the amount of pressure produced by your heart between beats) is between 90 and 99.

Dr. White thinks that what happens is that the doctor just fails to see mild hypertension as a significant problem in the vigorous person sitting across from him. "He thinks, 'Okay, this person is 40 and pretty healthy otherwise, with a blood pressure of 140/90,' " says Dr. White. "And he thinks that this isn't very serious. The patient thinks that he's healthy because he doesn't have something bad enough to get medicine for. But

Mistakes Patients Make
under Pressure

Nobody is blameless. And patients make mistakes, too. The two big ones in blood pressure treatment are both what doctors call compliance problems.

First, some people avoid making lifestyle changes. "The likelihood that a patient will comply long-term with nondrug therapy is pretty dismal," says William B. White, M.D., chief of the section of hypertension at the University of Connecticut Health Center in Farmington. "Somebody will be really great for four to six months—he'll lose weight, so his pressure will go down. You see him the next year and he's gained weight back and stopped exercising. The next thing you know, the pressure is back up. Then the physician is likely to resort to prescribing medications to control blood pressure."

Before you and your doctor reach that point, though, there are a few other tactics that you can try.

- Ask your health insurance provider or local hospitals and health groups where to find hypertension support groups.
- Look in your local newspaper for heart-healthy cooking classes. They're cropping up all over.
- Use a home blood pressure monitor regularly to get feedback on how well lifestyle changes are working for you.

mildly elevated blood pressure is likely to become even higher over time. So the patient's problem resurfaces five years later when his blood pressure is 160/110. During that interval, some damage has occurred, such as cardiac changes associated with blood pressure elevation or some kidney problems."

Dr. Gifford believes in very early intervention—when blood pressure is high-normal, or 130 to 139/85 to 89. "But doctors don't tend to make much fuss if blood pressure is 135 over 85. The message doesn't come across that it might be risky. And that's the time to get to it. There's really good evidence that you can prevent high blood pressure then, before it gets worse," he says.

Unless blood pressure is high—over 160/105, says Dr. Gifford—or it's complicated by a condition like diabetes, prompt treatment of choice

---

- Tap into the patient-support group on the Hypertension Network's high blood pressure Web site at http://www.bloodpressure.com.
- Join a health club or a gym. Or find a buddy to work out with.

A second common problem is not taking the medication. Sometimes, people don't take the drug that can help them because they regard even an aspirin with distrust. Often, it's because they're having side effects with one drug, which makes them dismiss all drugs in the blood pressure arsenal. "It's very difficult to convince people to take medication for the rest of their lives. Often, people feel well, so they tend not to take medication," says Harry Gavras, M.D., vice-chairman of the American Heart Association's Council for High Blood Pressure Research and chief of the hypertension and atherosclerosis section of Boston University Medical Center.

If the idea of taking a pill every day of your life turns you off, you need to do a little research on why it's so necessary. Ask your doctor to point you in the direction of information. If there are side effects that have understandably put you off pill taking, be aware that there are six very different classes of drugs for blood pressure and many medications in each class. "You really need to get on different medication. It shouldn't produce side effects," says Thomas G. Pickering, M.D., professor of medicine at the hypertension center at New York Hospital–Cornell Medical Center in New York City and author of *Good News about High Blood Pressure*.

means initiating lifestyle changes.

"Lifestyle changes are very important," says Dr. Gavras. "Your doctor should educate you to eat less sodium and lose weight and exercise with activities like walking. Just by decreasing sodium intake and losing weight, one-third of those with hypertension can control their blood pressures."

But doctors seem more at ease with drugs than with eating or exercise regimens, says Dr. White. "We have a much harder time educating patients about lifestyle changes. It's hard to implement because physicians don't have the time or the background information on how to educate patients during the short encounters that they have with them," he says.

So when doctors finally nab blood pressure at stage one, they often do so with medication. "When a doctor doesn't have time, it's easy to just say to the patient, 'You have high blood pressure—I'll give you a prescription,'" says Sheldon G. Sheps, M.D., chief of the hypertension division at the Mayo Clinic in Rochester, Minnesota. If you find yourself in that position, and your blood pressure is mild and uncomplicated, Dr. Sheps says, "Then it's alright for you to say, 'I've been reading that I might be able to help my blood pressure by losing 10 pounds, and I'd like to try that first. Is it okay? If it doesn't work in three months, I'll consider medication.'"

But if your blood pressure is high-normal and you'd like to take it down a notch even though your doctor seems unconcerned, ask him about lifestyle changes. "It's always a good idea to ask about ways to change your diet and exercise. I also think it's a good idea to ask if you should have a medical evaluation before you start an exercise program," says Dr. White. This precaution is especially recommended if you're middle-age and have been sedentary for years.

Here are the top lifestyle changes that experts recommend.

If you're overweight, lose some pounds. "You get the biggest bang for your buck right here," says Dr. Gifford. Even 10 pounds may be enough to give you the control that you need. Why is it so important? Extra fatty tissue makes your heart pump harder.

Control your salt intake. Give up table salt and cooking salt, advises Dr. Gifford. And rely more on fresh foods than salty, processed ones, he says. Half the folks who have high blood pressure are sensitive to sodium. Excess salt makes them retain water, which waterlogs blood vessels, narrows them, and makes the heart work too hard. (Talk to your doctor before making major dietary changes.)

Run for your life. Aerobic exercise has been shown to reduce the level of blood pressure if it's done for 40 minutes three times a week or more. The effect is greatest on the top (systolic) number. Aerobic activities include such things as walking, biking, and swimming. Whether or not poundage is a problem, working out tones the heart as well as the muscles, studies show. Weight training (when done properly—not holding your breath, avoiding prolonged gripping, and using weights that you can easily handle) can also reduce blood pressure.

Cut down on alcohol. Two drinks a day is the absolute maximum, experts say.

Stop smoking. It's *the* major risk factor for heart disease.

#4: Doctors Prescribe Too Many Drugs

"There's a tendency among physicians to just add blood pressure medications when one isn't working adequately, rather than to try substituting them," says Dr. Pickering. "Some medications really just don't work on particular patients. In those people it would make more sense to substitute something that does work, not pile one drug on top of another."

Part of the problem, he says, is that trying to find out whether a medication is working involves taking lots of blood pressure readings. But if you get only three readings at a doctor's visit, and you have only one visit every few weeks, it's difficult to get enough data to make a good decision on medication. If you're trying a series of drugs to see which is best, it's cumbersome and expensive to do it by going to the doctor every week.

One thing that you can do, Dr. Pickering says, is "self-monitor your blood pressure. It's economical and easy to tell if medication seems to be working by using a home monitor. Then you can phone in or fax in your readings. The doctor can get a feel for whether the stuff is working. It's a valuable way to assess medication."

#5: Doctors Don't Tell You about Timing

Strokes and heart attacks tend to occur early in the morning. Blood pressures tend to be high then, too. So it would make sense to take your medicine in the morning when it would do the most good. But many doctors don't talk about the best time to take blood pressure medication.

Even when they do, "medicines don't affect everybody the same," says Dr. Sheps. The rate at which your body absorbs medications may be different from your neighbor's. "And some medications need to be taken on an empty stomach," he says.

But you can double-check the timing yourself with a home monitor. "Take one reading in the morning after you get up and get ready for the day, but before breakfast," says Dr. Sheps. "Sit down for 5 minutes—read the paper or watch the news—and take your blood pressure seated. Take it again at the end of the day. Use the same sequence of letting your body settle down for 5 minutes. This tells you when your peaks and valleys are—in the morning or evening. Then your physician can adjust the timing of your medication."

Men's Health

Intriguing evidence suggests that slashing fat consumption and other dietary changes can slash your risk of developing prostate cancer.

Men over 40 take note: Scientists want to rewrite the battle plan against prostate cancer. The old plan featured two big guns—early detection and treatment. The new plan would add a weapon that until recently had been barely whispered in the world of prostate research: prevention through diet.

The hope that nutrition can actually deter prostate cancer as it does heart disease has spawned compelling research. And it seems to be coming at just the right time. More men now seem to be aware of the threat of this cancer than at any other time. The walnut-size gland that sits at the base of a man's bladder is finally getting some respect. This new awareness is due in part to some famous men, like Norman Schwarzkopf and Bob Dole, who have made no secret of their battles against prostate cancer.

"Prostate cancer is coming out of the closet," says William Fair, M.D., chief of urologic oncologic surgery at Memorial Sloan-Kettering Cancer Center in New York City. "Fifteen to 20 years ago, you couldn't even mention the word *prostate* in mixed company." Now we know that in sheer numbers there will be far more cases of prostate cancer this year than of breast cancer. One in five men will get prostate cancer in his lifetime. The highest risk is for men over 50, but younger men get prostate cancer, too.

The buzz about possibly preventing prostate cancer seems so tantalizing in part because treating it is not always so simple. The standard treatments—surgery, radiation, hormonal therapy, and cryotherapy—can often shrink tumors or effect cures. But sidestepping their side effects is not always easy. Can nutrition really make all this unnecessary—or at least far less likely? Can a knife and fork head off this men-only cancer before doctors have to step in?

The Trail of Clues

One of the first hints that diet might play a role in preventing prostate cancer came from studies of Japanese men, who generally eat more vegetables and less fat than most American men do. "Research revealed that although Japanese men get prostate cancer at the same rate as men in the United States, far fewer Japanese men die from it, because the cancer doesn't grow," says Moshe Shike, M.D., director of clinical nutrition at Sloan-Kettering. What's more, when Japanese men move to the United States (where diets differ from typical Japanese fare), their risks of faster-growing prostate cancers increase.

"These studies argue strongly for something in the environment that affects cancer risk," says Dr. Shike, "and the strongest environmental factor appears to be diet."

In fact, animal research led by Dr. Fair and Warren Heston, Ph.D., director of the George M. O'Brien Prostate Research Center at Sloan-Kettering, underscores the diet connection, especially the fat factor. They and their colleagues discovered that it was difficult to grow prostate tumors in

When Should You Start Screening?

The American Cancer Society recommends screening annually with a prostate-specific antigen, or PSA, test starting at age 50. (If you're African-American or have a family history of prostate cancer, talk to your doctor about starting your screening program earlier.) You should also start getting yearly digital rectal exams at age 40.

mice that ate low-fat diets. Their research also shows that growth of established tumors in mice slows when the fat that the animals eat is restricted.

Another strand of evidence also hints at a fat connection. If a man
eats too much fat, it has been shown that his testosterone level increases—
and increased testosterone, researchers say, may help stimulate the growth
of prostate tumors. So, through mechanisms that scientists haven't fath-
omed yet, it may be that too much fat in the diet increases prostate cancer
risk.

But fat isn't the only dietary factor linked to prostate cancer. There's
also soy. As Dr. Shike points out, Japanese men not only eat a diet that's up
to 20 percent calories from fat (as opposed to the 36 percent that the average American eats), they also eat a lot of soy—far more soy than American men. For Japanese men, tofu—curdled soy—is a way of life. In lab
tests researchers have uncovered an eye-opening interaction between
prostate cancer cells and soy.

"If we add soy protein in the medium in which the cells are growing, we markedly inhibit growth," says Dr. Fair. "In fact, most of the cells
die." Even better, if soy is fed to mice that have prostate cancer, tumor
growth slows down or stops.

Then there's the tomato connection. A study of 47,849 men, published in the *Journal of the National Cancer Institute,* has shown a link between high intake of tomatoes, especially tomato sauce cooked with a
little olive oil, and a lower risk of prostate cancer.

Compared with men who ate no tomato sauce, men who ate as little as two servings a week had a 34 percent reduction in risk for prostate
cancer. Though tomatoes alone were associated with lowering the risk,
tomato sauce had the strongest link.

"We theorize that this is because the cooking process and the oil in
the sauce seem to enhance absorption of lycopene," says Edward Giovannucci, M.D., Sc.D., assistant professor of medicine at the Harvard School
of Public Health. Lycopene is a carotenoid, one of the phytochemicals
found in produce that may contain anti-cancer agents. Keep in mind that
you don't need a lot of olive oil in the sauce to increase the absorption.

What You Can Do

Right now, no expert is ready to tell men that eating a certain way is
definitely going to prevent prostate cancer. But some researchers like Dr.

*Herbal*SOLUTION

Can Saw Palmetto Help?

A widely used plant extract used to treat benign prostatic hyperplasia (BPH)—enlarged prostate—comes from saw palmetto (*Serenoa repens*), a dwarf palm tree that grows in the southeastern United States and the Caribbean. The extract of the berry is used widely in Europe—in Germany, saw palmetto and other plant extracts are used to treat nearly 90 percent of BPH patients. Though many men have claimed that saw palmetto has helped them, the best research on the subject is inconclusive. But scientists do believe that the herb shows enough promise to continue the research.

Varro E. Tyler, Ph.D., Sc.D., former professor of pharmacognosy at Purdue University in West Lafayette, Indiana, and author of *The New Honest Herbal* and *Herbs of Choice*, advises any man who wants to try saw palmetto to first do two things: get a diagnosis (maybe it's BPH, maybe it's not) and discuss the herb with your physician. Saw palmetto seems to have no serious side effects, though in rare cases it can cause stomach upset. Effects of long-term use are unknown. "It's very much a matter of 'use at your own risk' because it's not an approved drug in the United States," says Dr. Tyler.

It's sold in supermarkets and health food stores as a dietary supplement, not as a drug, so there are no standards of quality. Dr. Tyler's tip is to read the label. It should say that it's standardized to contain 85 percent to 95 percent of fatty acids and sterols. The usual dose is 80 to 160 milligrams twice daily.

Keep in mind that taking saw palmetto can decrease prostate-specific antigen (PSA) test readings and can mislead you and your doctor into thinking that your prostate is cancer-free, says E. David Crawford, M.D., chairman of the division of urology at the University of Colorado Health Sciences Center in Denver.

If you choose to use this herb, stop taking it for at least 24 hours before and 24 hours after your scheduled PSA test, says David Bouda, M.D., assistant professor of oncology at the University of Nebraska School of Medicine in Omaha. Doing that will improve the accuracy of the test and may increase the chances of early cancer detection.

Fair are saying that for men who are at high risk for prostate cancer, eating the kind of diet suggested by existing cancer research may be a good bet, especially since the diet is already known to help prevent heart disease as well as other types of cancers. (Men's risks increase with age. Other risk factors include being African-American, having a family history of prostate cancer, or having an elevated PSA level.) Keep in mind that these dietary suggestions aren't meant to be substituted for medical treatment or screening. The guiding principles of this diet, then, are as follows.

Ditch the fat. "That's the single best recommendation we have," says Dr. Fair. To reach the 20 percent level used in the research, set a fat target. If you consume 2,000 calories per day, 400 of those calories can come from fat (2,000 × 20 percent = 400). And since there are 9 calories in each gram of fat, you can eat about 44 grams of fat per day (400 ÷ 9 = 44.4). This is your fat target. Depending on your weight and activity level, you may consume more or less than 2,000 calories a day; if so, adjust your fat intake accordingly.

A Guy's Guide to Smart Eating

You decide to give your prostate every possible break and switch to a low-fat diet that includes soy, tomatoes, and plenty of vegetables. But restaurants and ballparks may not be so accommodating to your new dietary goals. What's a guy to do?

Don't give up hope. Here are prostate-friendly alternatives for three difficult dining situations that you might find yourself in.

The luncheon. Meeting an important client for lunch? No problem. Head for your favorite Chinese restaurant but skip the sweet-and-sour fried shrimp. Instead, choose steamed vegetables with tofu (with sauce on the side) or try a vegetable-and-tofu stir-fry with a side of brown rice (ask them to go easy on the oil). Then later, for dinner, cut down on the fat, since stir-fry dishes tend to be a little greasy.

Boys' night out. You're playing cards with your buddies. Instead of greasy potato chips and high-fat dip, have baked tortilla chips and salsa.

Dinner for two. You've offered to cook for your significant other tonight, and you're out to impress. You can't miss with a hearty lasagna that packs a double whammy: tomato sauce and tofu.

Thanks to today's detailed food labels, it's easier than ever to calculate how much fat you're eating. And it's simpler than you think to find low-fat meals that taste great. Many magazines and cookbooks have good ideas on finding and creating low-fat, tasty meals and snacks.

Some little things can make a big difference in your fat intake. Eat less red meat, cut out fried foods, and switch to skim milk, and you'll make a big dent in your fat intake. Other tactics include using mustard instead of mayonnaise on your sandwiches, trying balsamic vinegar on your salads, and not buttering your bread.

Bring on the soy. Dr. Fair and others recommend at least 20 grams of soy a day. Don't worry; there's more to soy than just tofu, though that's a versatile source that you can add to salads, sandwiches, and stir-fry dishes. (Look for the low-fat variety, which gives you 6 grams of protein per ⅓ cup.) Other options include ready-to-eat soy breakfast cereal (25 grams of soy protein per ½ cup), low-fat or nonfat soy drinks (3 to 4 grams of protein per cup), and soybeans (15 grams per ½ cup of dried beans and 12 grams per ¼ cup of canned).

Go tomatoes. Get two or more servings of tomato sauce a week. Try pizza or pasta with tomato sauce or even lasagna made with nonfat cheeses. Just don't go overboard. "We don't want people to eat 10 pizzas a week just to get their servings of tomato sauce," says Dr. Giovannucci.

Round up the usual suspects. Some nutritional factors haven't yet been linked to a lower risk of prostate cancer but are known to reduce the risk of many other types of cancer. Experts agree that it just makes good sense to include these in any dietary defense against prostate cancer. These include the following:

- Eight or more servings of fruits and vegetables a day. That may sound like a lot, but when you consider that one carrot is two servings and a 6-ounce glass of fruit juice also counts as a serving, the points add up fast.
- Lots of dietary fiber. The standard recommendation is to work toward eating 25 to 35 grams of dietary fiber per day. Most people can handle this amount, as long as it's introduced into their diets a little at a time. Brans and beans are good bets. A high-fiber cereal can give you 13 to 15 grams per ½-cup serving. Legumes—such as lima beans or lentils, which have from 5 to 7 grams per ½-cup serving—are good sources, too.

Natural Weight Control

The secret of weight control isn't denial, experts say. In fact, savoring your favorite foods can actually help you enjoy the experience more and eat less.

Dean Ornish, M.D., really likes a food that might surprise you. No, make that shock you.

"Yes, I like chocolate," says the world-famous doctor who is the leading exponent of ultra low fat eating. "I'm healthy, my cholesterol is 130, I don't have heart disease, and I've been eating a low-fat vegetarian diet since I was 19. A little chocolate isn't going to hurt me."

The important phrase here is "a little." When Dr. Ornish says "a little," he really means it. And here's his secret: He indulges in food in a very focused way. . . a way that maximizes pleasure and minimizes quantity.

One Bite Goes a Long Way

The taste treat that thrills Dr. Ornish most deeply is a dark, bitter-sweet chocolate candy with a bit of caramel in the center. "One piece is bite-size," says Dr. Ornish, president and director of the Preventive Medicine Research Institute in Sausalito, California. "(It's) only the calorie equivalent of maybe a teaspoon of premium ice cream."

But Dr. Ornish makes the eating of just one bit of chocolate a great big party. . . for one. "I'm not talking to anyone and I'm not on the phone or reading," he says. "First, I look at it. Then, I close my eyes and smell it. I bite in slowly. I notice all the different flavors, the textures, and the way it feels going down my throat. I notice that the flavors occur at different times, almost like a symphony, in different parts of my mouth and throat. Then, there are the different aftertastes."

The whole encounter takes several minutes. "I do it two or three times a week," Dr. Ornish says. "And usually, I find that one is all I want. It's enough. The experience lingers."

Feed Your Head

There's a reason that we're revealing Dr. Ornish's deep, dark chocolate secret. He is one of many experts who believes that paying close attention to what you are munching on can help prevent overeating—whether you're indulging in a treat or sitting down for a whole meal.

"If you pay more attention to your food, you may enjoy it more. And the payoff is, you may be satisfied by eating less," says Thomas Wadden, Ph.D., director of the Weight and Eating Disorders Program at the University of Pennsylvania School of Medicine in Philadelphia.

Researchers have reached the same conclusion elsewhere. At the University of Massachusetts Medical Center's Stress Reduction Clinic in Worcester, for instance, psychologists teach people who come in with a variety of medical problems how to increase their awareness of themselves, their surroundings, and of the present moment. This way of thinking—which they call mindfulness—helps a person turn down the stressful thoughts that exacerbate medical problems, including overeating.

The very first lesson that is taught to everyone who comes to the clinic is called the Raisin Meditation. Interestingly, it's very similar to the way Dr. Ornish eats chocolate.

"Each patient is given two raisins. Then we take about 5 minutes to eat just one of them," explains Jon Kabat-Zinn, Ph.D., a mindfulness meditation expert at the clinic. "First, we examine the raisin. We feel its texture and notice its colors. We imagine the grapes growing on the vines, in the fields, the sun pouring on them; the rain falling; the people picking them. We smell the raisin. Then, with awareness of what the arms, lips, and teeth are doing, we slowly put the raisin in our mouths. We chew slowly, experiencing the taste with full attention. After swallowing, we even imagine our bodies being one raisin heavier. Then, patients eat the next raisin the same way."

Those two little raisins carry a powerful lesson, especially for the people who come for the clinic's eight-week compulsive-overeaters' program, says clinic psychologist Elizabeth Wheeler, Ph.D., who leads the program. "The patients invariably say that they've never eaten anything that slowly," says Dr. Wheeler. "They're really surprised by how much they enjoy it, how much they taste it, how different it is from the usual eating experience."

Four Minutes to Stop Overeating

"Many people who have food problems eat on automatic pilot," Dr. Wheeler says. "A lot of times, the only way they know that they've eaten is because the food is gone. That's not satisfying."

To short-circuit automatic-pilot eating all of Dr. Wheeler's patients learn a powerful mini-awareness exercise that they're instructed to use before, during, and after eating meals.

By setting aside a few minutes before, during, and after your meal for awareness exercises, you can reduce the likelihood of overeating. "This time helps people maintain some level of calmness, control, and choice," says Dr. Wheeler. "It helps take the whole eating process off automatic pilot."

Two minutes before the meal. Sit in your chair quietly. Take five or six long, deep breaths. Let yourself feel relaxed.

Weight-Loss Friends and Foes

A rose by any other name may smell as sweet, but 240 calories of apple is two times sweeter to your appetite-control system than 240 calories of ice cream. That's just one surprise from research conducted at the University of Sydney, Australia.

In the study students were asked to come in each morning and eat 240-calorie portions of a specific food. Then they rated their feelings of hunger or fullness every 15 minutes. At the end of two hours came the ultimate test of how satisfied the students really were: They were allowed to hit a buffet table and eat as much as they liked, while researchers took copious notes.

A number of foods were tested, and when the crumbs settled, it was very apparent that equal caloric portions of different foods do not equally satisfy hunger. Basing their ratings on a scale that assigned white bread an automatic score of 100, the researchers discovered that some foods are only half as satisfying as bread, while others are actually three times more filling. At the bottom of the Aussie list (in the middle of a grease stain) were croissants. With a rating of 47, they were barely more satisfying than air.

The star performer at the top of the scale was the not-so-modest potato. With a way-out-in-front rating of 323, it gives you the most bang for your caloric dollar, filling you up faster and on fewer calories than any other food tested.

Here's how foods rate when it comes to satisfying hunger pangs. Choosing a food from the top of the list (high satiety-index scores) can fill your stomach without loading you down with unwanted calories.

One minute before the meal. Turn your attention to the coming meal. This is like saying grace, but it needn't be religious. If you're with other people, you might like to hold hands around the table. Think about how your food is the product of sunlight, rain, earth, and other people's labor. Think about the work required to prepare and cook it. And appreciate the fact that it's going into your body to nourish you.

Midway through the meal. Take another minute. Stop eating and take five deep breaths. Sit quietly for just a moment. You might realize that you're not hungry anymore.

Ten minutes after you're finished eating. Take one more minute to

Food	Satiety-Index Score
Potato	323
Fish	225
Oatmeal	209
Orange	202
Apple	197
Pasta, whole-wheat	188
Beefsteak	176
Grapes	162
Popcorn	154
Cereal, bran	151
Cheese	146
Crackers	127
Cookies	120
Banana	118
French fries	116
Bread, white	100
Muesli	100
Ice cream	96
Potato chips	91
Peanuts	84
Candy bar	70
Doughnut	68
Cake	65
Croissant	47

do another series of five deep breaths. Focus on the physical sensations that the food may be causing in your body. Hopefully, most are pleasant. But if a food makes you feel not so good afterward, you may decide to eat less of it in the future, Dr. Wheeler says.

"Mindfulness makes a big difference," says Dr. Wheeler. "A lot of people start to say, 'I don't need to eat as much because I'm enjoying my food more.' Some patients start losing weight immediately—even, sometimes, people who didn't come to the clinic for overeating." Follow-up studies of patients suggest that a program built around mindfulness works. "Our patients significantly reduce symptoms of compulsive eating," Dr. Wheeler says. "They're less likely to eat when they're not hungry and less likely to eat beyond the point of fullness."

Diet Secrets of a Professional Eater

Eating beyond the point of fullness isn't a problem for Gail Vance Civille—which is a little surprising, given her job description. As president of Sensory Spectrum in Chatham, New Jersey, she is paid by food manufacturers to evaluate their products. In other words, she often spends her entire day looking at food, thinking about food, and, of course, tasting food.

Although you might expect that Civille has a weight problem, she doesn't. At "well over 50," she is slender and healthy.

"Part of it is that I just don't find myself overeating very often," Civille says. "I think the reason is that I get a lot of satisfaction from each eating experience. For me, each mouthful becomes an event."

While Dr. Ornish comes to his chocolate with the goal of maximizing sensual pleasure, and patients in Dr. Wheeler's program aim at total awareness of food, Civille sits down to the table with the intention of thinking about food as well as savoring it.

There's a parallel, she explains, between the way she eats and the way her son, a film student, watches movies. "When my son watches a film, he puts a lot more effort into it than I do—I just let the film pour into my eyes. You can tell that my son gets intense satisfaction from movies because he's analyzing them while he watches. Well, that's the way I am with my food. I'm thinking about it while I eat."

Civille believes that if we think more about the things that we're eating, we'll appreciate food more . . . and eat less. Anyone, she says, can make the most of food in the same way that she does.

"Whenever you eat, ask yourself, 'What am I perceiving? What texture? What flavors? Are they what I expected from this food?'" Civille suggests.

While the main point here is maximizing satisfaction, occasionally, says Civille, you'll learn, by concentrating, that you don't like a food as much as you thought you did. In fact, you might not even want to finish eating it.

If you were trained as a taster by Civille, the first place that she would send you to learn about flavor and aroma is the spice shelf in your own kitchen. "I tell my trainees, 'Go home, open your spices, and start smelling them.' That's how you start to learn more about flavor and aroma.

"For just one example, we should all learn the differences among cinnamon, cloves, coriander, ginger, cardamom, and nutmeg," she says. "But most of us don't have a clue what the differences are. If you make the effort, though, you can learn. Then, when you taste a food, you can analyze what spices or herbs you're detecting."

Give Yourself a Limit

There's clearly a lot to be said for paying attention to your food, Dr. Wadden says. "Still, for most people with weight problems," he cautions, "there's one essential step that must come before mindfulness can be effective. That step is portion control. You should set a limit for yourself ahead of time."

The right limit certainly depends on your individual energy needs. But to some extent you can let common sense be your guide. If it's chocolate you adore, for instance, check the calories and the fat content. Limit yourself to something reasonable—for a deluxe bonbon, that might be one piece. (If you've been advised by your doctor to avoid all saturated fats, you might select a treat such as one fat-free chocolate sorbet bar or one single-serving cup of fat-free chocolate-cherry yogurt.)

For your dream macaroni-and-cheese recipe it might be ½ cup. At a cocktail party, it might be three hors d'oeuvres—your favorites from whatever is offered. If you're setting limits for a whole meal, aim for about the same quantity of food that you'd find in a reduced-calorie frozen dinner.

*Herbal*SOLUTION

Herbs to Pare Off Pounds

Here are several herbs that have helped people control their weight, according to James A. Duke, Ph.D., a retired U.S. Department of Agriculture botanist and author of *The Green Pharmacy.*

- Plantain or psyllium (*Plantago*, various species). Plantain is the leafy plant; psyllium is the seed of the same plant. In one Italian study scientists gave 3 grams of plantain in water 30 minutes before meals to women who were seriously obese—at least 60 percent over their recommended weight. The plantain group lost more weight than a similar group of women who simply cut back in their diets, Dr. Duke says.

  Russians have found that the weight-loss effect of plantain and psyllium is related to the spongy fiber in the seed (mucilage) and also to specific chemicals in the leaves (polyphenols).

  The easiest way to take psyllium is to eat a teaspoon of seeds before each meal, Dr. Duke says. Just don't inhale dust from the seeds. It can trigger asthma attacks in people who are sensitive to it. In fact, if you have asthma, avoid the seed entirely, he warns.

- Chickweed (*Stellaria media*). This has quite a folk reputation as a "slimmer." Try adding this vegetable to your diet and see what happens, Dr. Duke suggests.

Maximize Satisfaction

Once you've set your portion size, then go for it. Squeeze every drop of pleasure you can from that food by eating it mindfully. Even if your treat is low in calories—a ripe mango or a bowl of home-cooked vegetable stew—by eating it mindfully, you'll make the pleasure of any food more intense. Here are more tips to maximize satisfaction, eat less, and not feel deprived.

Eliminate distractions. "I used to eat while I was watching TV or talking to someone," recalls Dr. Ornish. "I'd be paying attention to that instead of to what I was eating, so I could go through a whole meal and not

Some people eat it raw in salads. Some steam it and eat it like a vegetable. Here's a "Weed Feed Mixture" that's favored by Dr. Duke for swifter slimming. Mix chickweed, dandelions, evening primrose, nettle, plantain, and purslane. You can eat this mixture of fresh herbs raw in a salad. You can also cook them as greens—spiced up, perhaps, with a slimming hot sauce.

- Red chili pepper (*Capsicum*, various species) and other hot spices. In one experiment researchers at Oxford Polytechnic Institute measured the metabolic rates of people on a standardized diet, then added a teaspoon of red-pepper sauce and a teaspoon of mustard seed to every meal. The study showed that the hot herbs raised metabolic rates by as much as 25 percent.

If you're trying to lose weight, you get another benefit from eating spicy foods, Dr. Duke says. The hot spice stimulates thirst, so you drink more liquids. If you fill up on water instead of food, you'll obviously take in fewer calories and gain less weight.

So hot, spicy foods just might help you keep your weight down. One caveat, though: Many people use hot spices in barbecue sauces on high-fat foods, such as spareribs, hot dogs, and sausages. If you have a yen for barbecue sauce but want to skip the fat, try Dr. Duke's "Hotdoggone." To a hot dog bun, add barbecue sauce, prepared mustard, and onion. Leave out the dog. It sounds weird, but this concoction is surprisingly satisfying, Dr. Duke says.

even taste the food. Then I'd look down and the whole plate would be empty and I'd wonder, 'Who ate this?' When I began to focus on what I was eating, I enjoyed the food much more, and I was able to become aware when I had had enough."

Shut your eyes. It's the ultimate way to shut out distractions, says Civille. "I often do this when I'm eating. My children are always embarrassed; they would prefer that I not look like I'm having a séance with my food. But it's worth it," she says. "When you close your eyes, you turn off the other distractions. You can just enjoy the food and become intimate with it."

(continued on page 202)

Real Life Story

When her husband was transferred from Kentucky to Florida, Janis Blevins, at age 39, became so depressed that she quit her job, stopped going out, and began to binge on Big Macs. Within a few years, the 5-foot-3, 120-pound mother of two had gained 113 pounds and lost all hope of ever being thin again. But a chance encounter at her doctor's office and a library card helped Blevins turn her life around and slim herself down permanently.

"All of my life, I lived in a small rural town with my family nearby. Moving was really devastating for me. At 39 I felt like the rug was being ripped out from under me. Leaving my family and friends left me feeling empty, and food helped fill the void.

"To my surprise I loved Florida, but I couldn't stop gaining weight. For the next three years, I tried diet after diet, but they never worked. I'd deprive myself, lose 15 pounds, go off the diet, and gain back 20. Finally, at over 200 pounds, I became so frustrated with dieting that I threw away my scale and the smaller-size clothes I kept as an incentive to lose weight. I decided that I was going to be fat for the rest of my life.

"It wasn't until a year later, when a case of food poisoning sent me to the doctor, that I found hope. The doctor's receptionist told me her story about how she lost weight thanks to reading up on healthy eating, and it inspired me to try to lose weight one last time. But this time, I approached things differently. I knew from past experience that starving myself to lose weight wasn't the answer. There had to be a better way, and I was going to find it—at the library.

"I checked out books and took notes on everything from low-fat recipes to the proper way of doing a situp. At the same time, I ignored suggestions that I knew weren't realistic. Diets that relied on eating specific food combinations sounded silly. Exercise regimes that revolved around activities that I didn't like, such as aerobics and jogging, were out of the question, because if I didn't enjoy an exercise, I knew I wouldn't do it.

"After a month of research, I decided to put what I had learned into practice. I didn't start a diet—I started a new way of eating that wasn't about counting calories or starving. Instead, it was about eating plenty of nutritious, low-fat foods and then moving my body. I changed the way I cooked my favorite foods—a package of corn or a pot of mashed potatoes no longer got a half-stick of butter and a hefty shake of salt, but a modest dose of Molly McButter. I learned to snack on raw vegetables and pretzels instead of mixed nuts and cheese.

"My husband, Danny, supported me through it all. He willingly tried new foods (for us) like asparagus, broccoli, and cauliflower and spices like paprika, dill, and thyme. He didn't complain when nonfat cheese and yogurt replaced the high-fat versions, and he even brought home some low-fat recipes. Of course, there were a few flops—we ended up throwing out one fish dish—but on the whole we found a lot of wonderful new recipes.

To summarize her strategies: Blevins lowered the fat in the family meals, stopped eating red meat, and reduced sodium intake.

"But eating right was only half the story, and the easy half at that. Although I dreaded the Florida heat, I knew from everything that I had read that exercise was key to keeping the pounds off. So I started walking because it was an exercise I was likely to stick with. I'd go out in the mornings, when it was coolest and there weren't a lot of people around. At first it was terrible. After a block or two in the heat, I'd be red-faced and panting.

"I was embarrassed and I imagined that everyone who saw me was thinking, 'She's so big, why does she even bother?' Walking wasn't as bad when Danny came with me. Although he walked faster than I did, I felt more comfortable and confident with him. It wasn't just his kind words and praise that motivated me but also his actions. If it rained, he'd get out an umbrella or suggest that we walk at the mall. He really kept me going. His support even showed in the presents he gave me. For my 45th birthday he bought us both bikes. I almost cried. I was 45 years old, and I had never owned a new bike.

"Now, when I ride my bike or play any of the sports that I couldn't before, I feel like a kid again. I have so much energy. I'm out swimming, playing tennis, hiking, and taking long walks every chance I get. Of course, one thing has changed. Now when Danny and I go walking, he's the one who says, 'I can't keep up.' "

As a result of this program, Blevins lost 115 pounds in the span of two years. The resuling health benefits were lower blood pressure and cholesterol, fewer backaches, and discontinued ulcer medication. Blevins reports other benefits as well, including more self-confidence, more energy, and a healthier husband.

Involve your nose. Just before eating, Civille always takes a deep whiff of her food. "I try not to be too grotesque and put my nose in my plate," she says. "But by taking a moment to savor the smell of your food, you enhance the experience."

In fact, you may be fooling your brain into thinking that you've eaten more than you did, according to neurologist Alan Hirsch, M.D., director of the Smell and Taste Treatment and Research Foundation in Chicago. "The brain interprets the amount of food that you've smelled as food that you've eaten," he says. "By sniffing your food before you eat it, you get more of the aromatic molecules called the volatiles up into your nose. They are carried to the olfactory bulb behind the bridge of the nose, where a lot of flavor perception takes place. That may diminish appetite, so you eat less."

Slurp. In Japan, it's weird *not* to slurp your noodles. There, slurping signifies enjoyment—and that belief is based in biological fact. "Bringing air into the food aerates more of the volatiles, so more flavor reaches your olfactory bulb," Dr. Hirsch says. True, slurping isn't considered mannerly in this country. But at a table for one, in the privacy of your home, you may want to try this one. Think of it as a cross-cultural experience.

Chew a lot. Chewing your food for a long while has the same effect as slurping: transporting the volatiles up the nose to maximize flavor and reduce appetite, says Dr. Hirsch.

Warm it up. Warm foods have more flavor because, you guessed it, more of the volatiles are released. That's one reason that Civille usually warms up her leftovers. "If you eat ravioli out of the fridge, you won't be getting as much of a flavor hit as when you warm it up," she says. "When it's cold, you might end up eating more, looking in vain for the flavor experience."

Watch your appetite wane. Cultivate an awareness of the changes in your appetite during a meal. Specifically, as you eat, you not only become less hungry but food also doesn't taste as good to you as it did at first, according to Dr. Hirsch. "The first bite of a steak always tastes the best," he says. "By the end, you've saturated your olfactory receptor sties, and you might as well be eating horse meat." So if you're no longer hungry, and you're not savoring it, that's a really good time to stop.

Osteoporosis

We need all the help we can get to fend off osteoporosis, the brittle-bone disease that afflicts 20 million Americans— mostly women, but some men, too. Here's a special exercise prescription that can help all of us prevent it.

You've heard of exercise to condition your heart and build your muscles. But what about exercise to strengthen your bones? The right kind of workout can do just that. In fact, the latest research hints that certain kinds of exercise can not only help a woman protect herself against the bone loss that comes with aging but may even increase her bone mass in certain areas, as well.

Up to age 35, women's bodies act like smart investors if they follow a healthy lifestyle. That is, a healthy woman's body deposits more bone cells than it withdraws from the skeleton. But from then on, withdrawals become more frequent while deposits remain the same.

Once a woman is in menopause, those withdrawals escalate from a lack of estrogen. For too many women the balance sheet goes deep into the red, and osteoporosis is the result. And by the age of 50, a woman's lifetime odds of breaking a bone because of osteoporosis are almost one in two. Hip fractures are by far the most devastating consequence.

But no woman has to resign herself to nature's bookkeeping. There is plenty that you can do to deter or treat osteoporosis.

But if exercise is one of the weapons against this bone-thinning disease, how exactly should you use it? How much exercise is enough to help beef up your bones? And what kind of bone-building exercise is best for you?

Here's what top doctors in exercise and bone health have to say, along with their recommended workouts for maximum bone health.

Bone-Building Basics

How can a physical activity build bones? Two ways: impact and muscular contractions. Impact is the amount of force placed on a bone. When you step down from a curb, you're increasing the impact on your skeleton. This impact is greater than when you're walking on an even sidewalk. The skeletal impact is also greater when you leave the supermarket carrying bags of groceries than when you went in empty-handed. And any increased impact signals to the bones to get stronger by adding more bone mass.

Muscle contractions help build bones, too, because muscles are attached to bones. When muscles contract, they pull on bone. The bigger and stronger the muscles, the more they pull on bone. Researchers believe that the more the pull, the more the bone is strengthened.

Based on your everyday activities, your skeleton settles in at a level of bone strength capable of withstanding the impacts and muscle contractions that it's used to. So if you sit at a computer all day and regularly plop in front of the television after dinner, your bone strength will likely be lower than that of a waitress who's on her feet all day. In general, the more active you are, the stronger your bones are. "So you want to add as much weight-bearing physical activity to your daily life as you can," says Gail Dalsky, Ph.D., director of the exercise research lab at the University of Connecticut Health Center in Farmington.

But there's more to exercising your way to stronger bones than that. To really do it right, keep these tips in mind.

Zero in on specific bones. There's no one activity that builds all bones. "To strengthen a bone, you have to do an exercise or activity that specifically targets that bone," says Dr. Dalsky. So, for example, while jogging may give your spine a jolt of strength, it does little for your wrists.

Surprise your bones. Research suggests that bones are strengthened the most when they're subjected to forces that they're not used to, says Robert Marcus, M.D., professor of medicine and director of the aging study unit at Stanford University School of Medicine. For example, walking has always been an old standby in the fight against osteoporosis. But if you walk the same amount every day, day in and day out, your bones become accustomed to that level of activity. To stimulate an increase in bone density, you'd have to increase the amount of walking that you do—or increase the load on your bones when you do your regular walking routine.

Another good way to give your bones a little surprise is to add activities to your exercise routine that are out of the norm. If you always walk, for example, mix in some step aerobics, racquetball, or rowing.

Stay in motion. Building bone isn't like erecting a permanent building framework and then being done. Steel lasts for centuries; your

Weed Out Osteoporosis

If you're looking to consume less protein and more nutrients that help prevent osteoporosis, botanist James A. Duke, Ph.D., a retired U.S. Department of Agriculture botanist and author of *The Green Pharmacy*, suggests that you try these remedies.

- Dandelion (*Taraxacum officinale*). Dandelion shoots are a good source of boron, and boron helps raise estrogen levels. Dandelion also has more than 20,000 parts per million of calcium, meaning that just 10 grams (just under 7 tablespoons) of dry dandelion shoots could provide more than 1 milligram of boron and 200 milligrams of calcium. Dandelion is also a fair source of silica, which some studies suggest also helps strengthen bone.
- Pigweed (*Amaranthus,* various species). On a dry-weight basis pigweed leaves are one of our best vegetable sources of calcium, at 5.3 percent, Dr. Duke says. This means that a small serving of steamed leaves (⅓ ounce or ⅒ cup) provides a hearty 500 milligrams of calcium. Other good plant sources of calcium, in descending order of potency, include lamb's-quarter, broad beans, watercress, licorice, marjoram, savory, red clover shoots, thyme, Chinese cabbage (bok choy), basil, celery seed, dandelion, and purslane.

bones won't. "You have to continue your activity level long term to keep up the strength of bones," says Barbara Drinkwater, Ph.D., research physiologist at the Pacific Medical Center in Seattle. "On a practical level this means choosing activities that are fun and that you will keep doing on a regular basis, and adding variety so that you don't get bored."

Consider taking estrogen. No matter how promising the news is on exercise—with the right type of exercise, you may actually increase bone strength—estrogen still counts. There's really nothing like it.

"Women need to keep in mind that exercise and calcium are additions to estrogen," Dr. Dalsky states. "If a woman is postmenopausal or

(continued on page 210)

Pick a Bone–Toning Program

The kind of bone-building exercise Rx that you need depends on your menopausal status, personal risk factors, and bone density (as measured by dual-energy x-ray absorptiometry, or DEXA, a narrowly focused x-ray beam that is the most highly rated bone-testing method). Menopause presents its own risk to your bones because of a lack of estrogen. But premenopausal women may be at an increased risk of osteoporosis because of the following:

- A personal history of having already broken a bone as an adult from modest trauma. (For example, you broke your arm after falling from a standing height as opposed to breaking a bone in a car accident.)
- A family history of osteoporosis, that is, a mother, grandmother, or sister diagnosed with osteoporosis.
- Long-term use of steroid or antiseizure medications or overuse of thyroid medication (a blood test can determine whether you're taking too much now). If you've taken any medication for six months or more, ask your physician if the medication could have affected your bones, since there are other drugs that also cause bone loss.
- Hyperthyroidism (overactive thyroid).
- Interrupted menstrual history: Any loss of periods for six months or more with the exception of pregnancy. (This is often seen in

If You Are . . .

Premenopausal

Without risk factors

With risk factors and DEXA T-score of:
    +1.0 and above

    -1.0 to +1.0

    -1.0 to -2.5

highly trained but underweight athletes, in women with eating disorders, or during times of emotional stress.)
- Hysterectomy prior to menopause with removal of ovaries and without replacement of estrogen. Loss of estrogen, whether from natural menopause or surgically induced menopause, is likely to trigger rapid bone loss in most women.
- Any period or restricted mobility for six months or longer, especially if it occurred in adolescence.

If you're premenopausal and have one or more of these major risk factors or if you have already gone through menopause, you need to have your bones checked with a bone-mineral density test using DEXA. (To help find a bone-testing facility near you, contact the National Osteoporosis Foundation at (800) 464-6700.) The results of your test will be expressed in standard deviations, or SDs, called a T-score.

+1.0 and above = strong bones

-1.0 to +1.0 = borderline bone strength

-2.5 to -1.0 = low bone strength

-2.5 and below = osteoporosis

With that information, you're ready to get your exercise prescription. The following recommendations—based on experts' assessments of available data—should help you figure out what's best for you.

Your Prescription Is . . .

Aerobic Activity (3 hr. per week)	Weight Training Sessions per Week (1/2 hr. each)*
jumping rope, running/jogging, aerobics, hiking, racquetball, tennis, volleyball	2–3
jumping rope, running/jogging, aerobics, hiking, racquetball, tennis, volleyball	2–3
low-impact aerobics, cross-country skiing, downhill skiing, rowing, square dancing, walking	2–3
low-impact aerobics, cross-country skiing, rowing, square dancing, walking	3

Pick a Bone-Toning Program—Continued

If You Are ...

Premenopausal—Continued

With risk factors and DEXA T-score of:
-2.5 and below

Postmenopausal

Taking estrogen and DEXA T-score of:
+1.0 and above

+1.0 to -2.5

-2.5 and below

Not taking estrogen and DEXA T-score of:
+1.0 and above

+1.0 to -2.5

-2.5 and below

* Seek the advice of an exercise professional to avoid injuring weak bone.

Your Prescription Is...

Aerobic Activity (3 hr. per week)	Weight Training Sessions per Week (1/2 hr. each)*
low-impact aerobics, cross-country skiing, cross-country ski machine, rowing, square dancing, walking, ballroom dancing, stairclimber, bicycling, swimming, water exercise	3*
jumping rope, running/jogging, aerobics, hiking, racquetball, tennis, volleyball	2–3
low-impact aerobics, cross-country skiing, rowing, square dancing, walking	2–3
low-impact aerobics, cross-country skiing, cross-country ski machine, rowing, square dancing, walking, ballroom dancing, stairclimber, bicycling, swimming, water exercise	3*
jumping rope, running/jogging, aerobics, hiking, racquetball, tennis, volleyball	3
low-impact aerobics, cross-country skiing, rowing, square dancing, walking	3
low-impact aerobics, cross-country skiing, cross-country ski machine, rowing, square dancing, walking, ballroom dancing, stairclimber, bicycling, swimming, water exercise	3*

amenorrheic (missing her periods), she needs to understand that calcium and/or exercise cannot prevent the bone loss that results from the estrogen deficiency of menopause or amenorrhea."

Of course, not all women can take estrogen or are comfortable taking the hormone. These women may consider one of the new bone-building drugs currently available, like alendronate or nasal-spray calcitonin.

But just as exercise can't fully substitute for estrogen, estrogen is no substitute for exercise if you want to go to the max for your bones. Research indicates that, while estrogen may be enough for women to maintain bone mass, only with the addition of exercise can women rebuild any of the bone that they may have lost.

In one study, published in the *Journal of Bone and Mineral Research*, 20 women who had undergone hysterectomies, producing surgical menopause, were split into two groups: one taking estrogen alone and the other taking estrogen while going through a program of weight training three times a week. The estrogen-alone group maintained the strength of spine and radius (the bone on the thumb side of your forearm). But in the estrogen-plus-exercise group spine density increased 8.3 percent and radial density increased 4.1 percent.

Let's be clear about the bone-exercise connection. Any physical activity can help maintain bone, if you use it to put new stresses on your bones. But some exercises may be better than others to boost bone mass.

It's important to remember, too, that some of the best bone-builders can be hard on the joints. Also, if you already have osteoporosis, some activities may increase your risk of fracture. So check out the guidelines on page 206 that apply to you and talk with your doctor before jumping into a new bone-building exercise program.

If you are vulnerable to bone loss in certain areas of your skeleton, it may be possible to give yourself an edge there. Some exercises are good at specifically targeting bones in fracture zones or those areas where osteoporosis hits hardest—the spine, hips, and wrists.

The best news is that one type of exercise—resistance training—may actually increase bone density in certain areas of the skeleton. It's already known that virtually any kind of weight-bearing exercise may at least slow the overall loss of bone. One of the studies showing specific-area increases through exercise was done by Miriam Nelson, Ph.D., and her colleagues at the U.S. Department of Agriculture Human Nutrition Research Center on Aging at Tufts University in Boston. The study put postmenopausal women from ages 50 to 70 who were not taking estrogen through a one-year program of resistance training for two days a week, 40 minutes a session. Those who did five different resistance-training exercises maintained total body-bone density, while those who didn't participate tended to lose bone density. But also, those in the exercise group, on average, gained bone density in the hip and spine.

"One of the most important outcomes from this study," says Dr. Nelson, "is that women greatly improved their strength—some got really strong—and their balance. When you consider that falls are the number one cause of fractures, especially hip fractures, you can see how important that improved balance really is."

Resistance training also may have the ability to target an area that few other activities can: the wrists and forearms. This is important because the wrists are likely to be the first fracture sites in women who develop osteoporosis. Racquet sports like tennis can increase wrist and forearm density only in the arm used.

If you have never worked out with weights before or have osteoporosis or weak bones, get some advice from a physiatrist, sports medicine doctor, or certified personal trainer.

Be Wary

Here are a few cautions for anyone with osteoporosis or weak bones. Anterior loads—holding weights out in front of you—can be dangerous. That's because they put a particular stress on your spine that can lead to compression fractures. Also, abdominal exercises like crunches or situps should be avoided until you see your doctor, since they can also lead to compression fractures. So, too, should exercises involving forward flexion of the spine (bending forward from a seated or standing position).

Also, for people with osteoporosis it's important to not only strengthen bones but also to improve balance, coordination, and muscle strength so that they lower their risk of toppling over. Besides resistance training, some activities not known for building bone, such as tai chi (a combined form of dance and karate), stationary bicycling, and water aerobics, may be helpful in improving balance, coordination, and muscle strength. Keep in mind that for many women with osteoporosis there remains an opportunity to regain some bone strength. And certainly, there's much that can be done to slow any further loss of bone.

Skin Problems

On the average most women have about 20 square feet of skin covering their bodies. Here's how to keep every inch of it in tip-top form.

So, you've let your skin regime slide. That doesn't mean that your skin needs to resemble the pallid gray of the Addams family complexions.

But to get dewy, young-looking skin, you may have to start with the foundation. In fact, you might have to try a new one. "Unfortunately, using the wrong foundation or applying the right one incorrectly can add years to your face," says Laura Geller, a celebrity makeup artist in New York City. Here's Geller's advice.

- Choose the right color. Test it on your jawline in natural, not fluorescent, light to see how it matches your skin tone. If there's no discernible difference, it's the correct shade. Too much orange can make you look older; too light a shade can leave you looking pale, tired, and drawn.
- Stick with a foundation that is rich in oil, if your skin is dry.
- Start with a moisturizer (preferably one with a sun protection factor). Moisturizers make it easier to apply and blend foundation. Use a sponge for even distribution, keeping in mind that less is more.
- Don't apply foundation on your neck; it emphasizes wrinkles.
- Over your foundation use a light dusting of translucent face powder. This sets the foundation, giving your skin an even, youthful tone. But don't overdo it, especially around wrinkles, because powder can collect in these lines and exaggerate them.

"If you spend 5 minutes in the morning and 5 at bedtime on a simple skin-rejuvenation plan, you can begin to see more glowing skin in only one week," says Fredric S. Brandt, M.D., clinical associate professor of dermatology at the University of Miami School of Medicine in Coral Gables, Florida.

What dewy skin needs is a three-step process.

Step 1: Cleanse

Cleansing sounds like a no-brainer, but doing it correctly can mean the difference between a complexion that looks rejuvenated and one that's

*Herbal*SOLUTION

Old Remedies Prevent New Wrinkles

Many commercial moisturizers are sold with the claim that they restore soluble collagen and rejuvenate the skin, allowing skin cells to absorb more fluid and banishing wrinkles, says James A. Duke, Ph.D., a retired U.S. Department of Agriculture botanist and author of *The Green Pharmacy*. But before you spend a fortune on any of these products, he suggests trying these natural approaches to prevent wrinkles.

- Horse chestnut (*Aesculus hippocastanum*) and witch hazel (*Hamamelis virginiana*). Japanese scientists tested 65 plant extracts and found seven that showed sufficient antioxidant activity to have potential against wrinkles, Dr. Duke says. But the researchers singled out horse chestnut and witch hazel as the best. Both of these are strong antioxidants. Soothing and astringent salves containing these herbs are available at health food stores.
- Rosemary (*Rosmarinus officinalis*). Another potent antioxidant, rosemary was identified by Japanese researchers as a promising wrinkle preventive and treatment. Use it as a culinary spice or make a tea with a teaspoon or two of crushed, dried leaves, Dr. Duke suggests.
- Sage (*Salvia officinalis*). Along with horse chestnut, witch hazel, and rosemary, sage was another common herb identified by Japanese researchers as a promising wrinkle preventive and treatment, though somewhat less effective. Use it as a culinary spice or try using a teaspoon or two of crushed, dried leaves to make a tea.

beyond ruddy. Your goal is to wash away makeup, dirt, and other potentially pore-clogging materials without stripping your skin of its protective barrier. Harsh cleansers can leave your skin more sensitive to everything—exfoliating ingredients, fragrances, and even the environment itself. "For the face I recommend very mild soaps, such as Basis, Dove, or glycerine soaps or a nondrying cleanser like Cetaphil," says Dr. Brandt. If your skin is sensitive, use fragrance-free products.

Step 2: Exfoliate

Before you can have a glowing complexion, the dead skin cells that leave you looking ashen must be removed. That's the job of exfoliation, and it can reveal skin that looks brighter and healthier, says Dr. Brandt. "Exfoliation even seems to stimulate collagen production and helps prevent clogged pores." What else can you ask for?

Well, a little simplicity might be good. There's a wealth of choices in the exfoliant arena. The broad categories are mechanical and cosmetic exfoliants. Mechanical means that you're rubbing off dead skin cells, and you can do that with a loofah, a face cloth, or with cleansing grains (sandlike particles in a cream, lotion, or gel that have an abrasive action on your skin). Cosmetic exfoliation means that an ingredient in your cosmetic product chemically loosens dead skin cells, allowing them to be washed away.

As a rule of thumb, mechanical exfoliators are best reserved for your body, while the chemical exfoliators are terrific for your face. If you're headed for mechanical exfoliation (which, by the way, you can also do with a mesh facial sponge, or Buf-Puf), "gentle" is your mantra.

Cosmetic exfoliation is a little more complicated as there are numerous nonprescription products currently begging to be next to your sink, usually in the form of glycolic acid (an alpha-hydroxy acid) or salicylic acid. Unfortunately, there's no way to know which is best for you until you try them. You may want to apply one to a small patch of skin first to see how your skin reacts. Always follow label directions. Consult a dermatologist if you think that you need a prescription exfoliant. There are several forms—glycolic acid, salicylic acid, tretinoin (Retin-A and Renova). Your dermatologist can help you decide which is best for you. (Some should not be used if you're going to be in the sun.)

Step 3: Protect

A word to the skin savvy: Exfoliators, especially prescription-strength chemical exfoliants, leave your skin very susceptible to sun damage. (Dead cells are actually somewhat of a sunblock.) That means that your complexion is doomed unless you wear a sun protection factor, or SPF, of at least 15.

If you use a moisturizer, however, sun protection may be taken care of, since more cosmetic companies are including sunscreens in their moisturizers. So if you choose a moisturizer to keep your newly luminous face looking refreshed, you can get two bonuses in one by selecting a brand that also has sunscreen.

Sleep Deprivation

An erratic sleep schedule, the most common casualty of shift work, can lead to a host of medical problems. Here's an hour-by-hour plan to help those on the graveyard shift live healthier lives.

We are creatures of the light. We sleep by night, awake with the sun, and go about our business during the day. As the sun slides into the west, our bodies begin to wind down in preparation for sleep and the rest that we need.

That's how it works for most of us. But not for all. One in five Americans lives on the other side of the clock, as a shift worker. These people sleep by day and toil at night to keep factories humming, hospitals in operation, and increasingly, to provide 24-hour services such as all-night supermarkets to an economy that never sleeps.

If you've never worked the night shift, you might think that adjusting to it would be simple enough—something that might take a few days to get used to. Nothing could be further from the truth. "Human beings are built to be daytime creatures. It's hard-wired into our circuitry," says Timothy Monk, Ph.D., D.Sc., professor of psychiatry at the University of Pittsburgh School of Medicine.

Even those who choose night work don't fully appreciate what they're up against, namely a powerful inner timing mechanism that regulates sleep and wakefulness and governs a daily ebb and flow of body chemicals. The body's internal clock is reset each day by the rising sun and evening darkness, creating a natural cycle called a circadian rhythm. "When you deliberately try to shift the sleep/wake cycle, it's like having a symphony with two conductors, each one beating out a different time," says Dr. Monk. "Your delicate internal rhythm goes haywire."

Making the Best of It

Part of the prescription for good sleep doubles as a prescription for good health. Fortunately, scientists today understand the body's natural rhythms better than ever before, and their search points to some helpful ways to get a good day's sleep. Here's a step-by-step plan to ensure that you have your best chance of getting it.

Before Work

Take sleep seriously. This may seem obvious, but many night-shift workers stagger home, turn on the TV, and fall asleep on the couch. It's no wonder they feel terrible when they wake up. "You need to treat sleep as a precious and fragile thing," says Dr. Monk. This requires some extra planning—yes, and extra hassle—that a night sleeper doesn't have to deal with.

- You will need to prepare a quiet room. Put dark, heavy drapes on the windows or at least tack up layers of black plastic garbage bags to block out sunlight. You may even want to place a strip of black tape over your alarm clock's liquid crystal display if you find that it's too bright.
- Put out the do-not-disturb sign. "Social custom makes it wrong to visit at 3:00 in the morning. But few people would think twice about visiting a night-shift worker at 3:00 in the afternoon," says Dr. Monk. Inform your friends of the hours that you keep and ask them not to disturb you. Put a sign on your door that says, "Quiet, shift-worker sleeping."
- Turn your thermostat down to a "night" setting of 65° to 68°F before you leave home for work. That way, the house will be cooler when you get home, which many people find more conducive to sleeping.

Take a nap. Can't sleep for more than 4 to 5 hours in the morning following your night shift? Schedule a nap for the afternoon, when a natural lull occurs. If you've managed 5 to 6 hours of sleep in the morning, your afternoon nap should be 15 to 45 minutes long. If you were only able to get 3 hours of sleep in the morning, go ahead and nap for about 2 hours in the afternoon. But, in general, napping longer than an hour may leave you groggy.

Exercise in the afternoon. Many people like to exercise in the morning, before other activities begin to encroach on their time. But that can be confusing, if not simply bad, advice for night-shifters. Exercising when you get home from a nighttime job will only make it more difficult for you to fall asleep. Instead, schedule your exercise for when you wake. And try to exercise outdoors if you can. That way, the sunlight may help shift your body clock into morning mode, making it easier to stay alert through the night.

There's also evidence that regular aerobic exercise may help you adapt to night-shift work better by shifting your circadian rhythms to match your sleep/wake schedule. The scientific research suggests that you need to exercise five times a week in order to successfully shift your circadian rhythm. That amount of exercise (at least) is recommended for preventing heart disease and overstuffed waistlines.

At Work

Enlighten your load. Exposure to bright light at night will help shift your body to day mode, especially when you avoid morning sun by wearing dark glasses on your drive home. In studies workers who sat under bright lights for 30 minutes to 2 hours between midnight and 4:00 A.M. were more alert and had better daytime sleep. Plus, they slept 2 hours longer. Some forward-thinking companies are hip to this new research and have installed bright light fixtures where their night-workers toil. Great, but you say that your boss is still living in the Dark Ages? Well, then you might have to take things into your own hands. Purchase a special high-intensity light box and give your body a dose before going to work or during your breaks.

Don't drink coffee after midnight. That goes for tea and cola, too. Caffeine stays in the body for 6 hours, says Scott Campbell, Ph.D., director of the Sleep Laboratory at the department of chronobiology at New York Hospital–Cornell University Medical College in New York City. It can interfere with sleep and also cause indigestion. His advice to night-shifters is to "have no more than 2 cups during your shift—the last one no later than midnight." (If you're a heavy coffee drinker now, phase down slowly. Cutting back too rapidly could produce caffeine withdrawal symptoms. And it's hard to sleep when you're nauseated and have a headache.)

It's 3:00 A.M. Do you know where your chicken is? Try eating your biggest meal during your night shift's lunch hour. This will re-

*Herbal*SOLUTION

Soothing Potions
for the Sleep-Deprived

Pharmaceutical sedatives work, but they can become addictive, and they interfere with natural sleep cycles, says James A. Duke, Ph.D., a retired U.S. Department of Agriculture botanist and author of *The Green Pharmacy*. So you won't be surprised to learn that he prefers the following natural alternatives.

- Melissa (*Melissa officinalis*). Also known as lemon balm, melissa is endorsed by Commission E as both a sedative and stomach-soother. (Commission E is the body of scientists that advises the German government about herb safety and effectiveness.) The sedative action is attributed largely to a group of chemicals in the plant called terpenes. Several other herbs are better endowed with some of these chemicals—juniper, ginger, basil, and clove—but none of them has the mix that melissa contains, and none of them has melissa's reputation as a bedtime herb, Dr. Duke says.

  He suggests trying a tea made with 2 to 4 teaspoons of dried herb per cup of boiling water.

duce your temptation to snack during the wee hours of the night.

And you should snack only strategically. Night-shift workers often face long hours of boredom. One way to pass the time is to eat. Unfortunately, the snack cart or vending machines rarely offer healthful choices. Make a point of bringing vegetables, fruits, low-fat yogurts, or air-popped popcorn to work with you.

Coffee-break a sweat. Instead of reaching for a cup of joe during your break, walk a few flights of stairs or stroll around your workplace. The benefits are twofold: You burn calories instead of consume them, and a study showed that workers who are allowed to take 20-minute exercise breaks report improved alertness—even at 4:00 A.M., when the body normally begins feeling sleepy.

- Valerian (*Valeriana officinalis*). A tea made with 1 to 2 teaspoons of dried valerian root shortly before bedtime will promote sleepiness, according to Commission E. In fact, the commission considers the tea so safe that it also endorses drinking it up to several times a day to relieve restlessness, anxiety, and nervousness.

  Valerian has a fairly rank aroma and taste. If its earthiness is not to your liking, you can always opt for capsules instead.

  In the United Kingdom, there are more than 80 over-the-counter sleep aids containing valerian. Why? Because it works. In one study a combination of 160 milligrams of valerian and 80 milligrams of lemon balm extracts brought on sleep as well as a standard dose of one of the drugs in the Valium family of pharmaceuticals (benzodiazepines), according to Dr. Duke. Unlike prescription sleep or anxiety medications, valerian is not considered habit-forming, nor does it produce a "hangover," as do medications in the Valium group, he says.

  Some naturopaths suggest that you treat insomnia by drinking valerian root about 30 minutes before retiring. Others suggest taking 150 to 300 milligrams of a standardized extract (0.8 percent valeric acid).

On Your Way Home

You have it made in the shade. Wear sunglasses to shade your eyes from the morning sun. In a study led by Dr. Eastman, night-workers who put on welder's goggles for the trip home found it easier to sleep and slept an average of 2 hours longer. The reason was that the goggles kept sunlight from cueing the body that it was morning. No one is suggesting that you drive around wearing welder's goggles, of course, but a pair of aviator glasses might help bring you in for a smoother descent to the land of dreams.

Bypass the diner. You can smell the bacon and hash browns halfway down the block. But don't turn into the parking lot of that diner. Eating a big meal at the end of your day—especially a traditional breakfast-type meal—signals your body that it's morning. And you'll have trouble getting to sleep. Also, eating heavy meals before you hit the sack may cause indigestion, not to mention weight gain over time.

At Home

Go to bed right away. Avoid the temptation to do chores, write out checks, or watch TV. Instead, wind down with a book, then go to bed quickly. Sleep specialists say that this is less disruptive to your body clock than staying up in the morning and sleeping in the afternoon.

Blot it out. Wear earplugs to dampen the daytime noises. Turn off the telephone ringer and disconnect the doorbell. Some people find that it helps to buy a white-noise machine, which emits a low, steady tone that masks other sounds. Others use recordings of the sounds of waterfalls or ocean waves to soothe them into slumber.

Avoid using sleep inducers. Probably the worst thing that you can do is drink yourself to sleep. Alcohol interferes with REM sleep, which is key to getting good rest. And though a drink may help you fall asleep faster, it also wakes you up sooner.

Melatonin supplements are all the rage these days for people looking for a little pill to help them sleep, beat jet lag, and reset their body clocks. These pills are a synthetic version of natural melatonin, a sleep-inducing chemical produced in the brain and released during the hours of darkness. Research has shown that melatonin may help shift your body clock to a night setting, so taking this supplement could be helpful in adapting to the first few days of night-shift work. But Dr. Monk warns that no studies have been done on the safety of melatonin supplements for long-term use.

Use sleeping pills wisely if you use them at all. One legitimate use of sleeping pills, says Dr. Campbell, might be to help rotating shift-workers sleep following their first day back on the night shift. Still, most experts have mixed feelings about chemical sleep aids: "The problem with sleeping pills is not so much physical addiction—they've worked on that. But they have a huge risk of psychological addiction," says Dr. Campbell. "You take it that first night, you sleep well, and you think, 'Why don't I do that every night of my night shift?'"

Make a Switch

Even if you follow the above advice, you may still find that working the night shift is not getting any easier. "Somewhere in their late thirties to mid-forties, many people just hit the wall," says Dr. Monk. Scientists don't understand exactly why aging makes us less adaptable to night-shift work, but in one study the sleep disruption was twice as bad in middle-age workers as in young workers.

Perhaps the best remedy for those whose bodies have trouble coping is to find work on the day shift. It's a healthier lifestyle in the long run. The disruptive patterns of the night shift put the body in a constant state of stress, which doctors believe causes the release of stress hormones that raise blood pressure and cholesterol levels. Over time this can take its toll: A study of nurses found that heart disease risk increased by nearly 50 percent in those who worked more than six years on the night shift. "You need to put this risk in perspective," says study leader Ichiro Kawachi, Ph.D., assistant professor at the Harvard School of Public Health. "It's not nearly as significant as smoking all your life or a sedentary lifestyle or a high-fat diet. Still, our research suggests that it's a good idea not to work nights for more than six years."

Finally, go easy on yourself if you're having trouble adjusting to the night shift. "The problem lies in your body," reminds Dr. Campbell. "It's not a personal failing."

Stress

We can't put brakes on the outside world. But to put the brakes on stress, there are many ways we can slow ourselves down, doctors say. Here's how to stop your lifestyle from gobbling up your energy.

When Sally's alarm goes off at 6:00 A.M., she steps onto a treadmill. It's a peculiar machine with limited options. No "reduce speed" button. No "pause." In fact, its nightmarish tendency is to speed up, racing faster and faster. For many of us, the treadmill is called life.

Don't say that you weren't warned. Virtually all of us have heard older folks complain that as the years pass, time seems to pick up momentum like a boulder barreling downhill. And the gathering momentum makes our lives seem more stressful—which, in turn, can hurt our health, doctors say.

Psychologists suggest that our perception of how time flies is, in part, related to the way that we perceive the span of a lifetime. "At age 5, a year is one-fifth of a whole lifetime; by age 50, it represents just one-fiftieth of your vast past. Still, this doesn't explain why so many of us lead lives greased for maximum speed, regardless of our ages.

Blame it in part on technology, says Stephan Rechtschaffen, M.D., author of *Time Shifting*. Technology allows us to perform endless tasks at speeds unthinkable in prior generations. Jets reduce long journeys to short junkets. Faxes cut mail time from days to minutes. And computers can process reams of information in a nanosecond (that's a billionth of a second).

"Thirty years ago, the promise of technology was that it would stretch our time for relaxation, being with families, and petting the dog," says Michelle M. Weil, Ph.D., clinical psychologist and partner with Byte Back Technology Consultation Services in Orange, California. Instead, we increasingly find that our time is shrinking.

"The problem is that we've simply developed the expectation that we can do more and more things in less and less time," says Dr. Rechtschaffen. And as we expand our to-do lists and cram our appointment calendars, the rhythm of our lives speeds up. With that enhanced speed comes exaggerated expectations—which accumulate to make our lives infinitely more stressful.

Rhythms and You

As human beings, we naturally respond to the rhythms of what's around us, Dr. Rechtschaffen continues. Studies have shown, for example, that our gestures, facial expressions, and speech patterns synchronize when interacting with others. Listen to a colleague chattering away and pretty soon you, too, are talking in fast-forward.

"We need a mutual framework of timing so that one person doesn't zig while the other person zags," says Frederick Erickson, Ph.D., director of the Center for Urban Ethnography (the observational study of human culture in everyday life) at the University of Pennsylvania in Philadelphia.

Similarly, without even knowing it, you synchronize with other signals in your environment. Drive through Manhattan during rush hour or

*Herbal*SOLUTION

Cool Out with This Tincture

If stress is a way of life for you, stay as far away as you can from recreational drugs, coffee, and tobacco, suggests Kathi Keville, director of the American Herb Association and author of *Herbs for Health and Healing*. In addition, try this herbal path.

- Kava kava (*Piper methysticum*). Kava kava lives up to its reputation of promoting peace and harmony among people, Keville says. In Polynesia, kava kava tea is used to induce relaxation, restful sleep, and a sense of mild euphoria. Here's a simple version of what Keville calls her Cool Out Tincture that should help you unwind.

  Combine 1 teaspoon each tinctures of valerian, rhizome, licorice root, Siberian ginseng root, kava root, and California poppy (if available). Take as needed during emergencies, up to 1 teaspoon per hour. Otherwise, take $^1\!/_2$ to 1 dropperful a day as a general relaxing aid.

step into a busy hospital emergency room. Chances are that your body will pick up the rhythm of the moment and send your pulse racing.

Consider, also, the many modern-day signals—like the red blinking light of a telephone answering machine or the beeping of e-mail—designed to arouse a sense of urgency, says Dr. Rechtschaffen. "A pager beeps very quickly. It says, 'Answer me, fast!'"

It's not that a fast pace is all bad. Speed can be exhilarating, like a roller-coaster ride. The problem occurs when you get so habituated to the fast track that you have difficulty downshifting even when the environment does. Or when it's bedtime and your mind is still buzzing with work. Or when you tote a laptop and cell phone along on vacation. Or when you run into an old friend and think, "Hurry up, tell me what's on your mind. I have things to do."

When the human pace is chronically breakneck, the primitive mechanism that prepares us to respond quickly—the so-called fight-or-flight response—gets abused. The result: mind- and body-ravaging stress.

Cultivating a Kinder Pace

Of course, we can't put the brakes on the external world. But we can slow ourselves down. "With practice we can develop the power to stop at any moment and change the rhythm of whatever we're doing, no

Silence the Din

Several studies have linked noise to increased stress. Noise has also been linked to high blood pressure, heart disease, mental health problems, and learning disorders.

"Most research deals with loud noise, but there's reason to believe that stress levels are affected by incessant noise, too," says Shirley Thompson, Ph.D., noise expert and epidemiologist at the University of South Carolina, Columbia. Perhaps the most detrimental effect of noise is its effect on the quality of life.

"When our days are full of TV, radio, and other chatter, noise squeezes out the silence in which to think, reflect, and find meaning in who we are and what we do," says Bruce Davis, Ph.D., psychologist and author of *Monastery without Walls: Daily Life in the Silence*. Excess noise clutters the mind like excess papers clutter a desk. You spend all day sifting through the chaff rather than focusing on what's important.

Silence offers reflective time to clear the clutter. "If we don't stop occasionally and look at where we've been and where we're going, we end up going round and round in circles," says Jeffrey A. Kottler, Ph.D., professor of counseling and educational psychology at the University of Nevada, Las Vegas, an expert on solitude, and author of *The Language of Tears*. "We rarely end up being where we really want to be in life."

When there's no pause in the input, our heads get filled with the voices and opinions of others—be it parents, friends, or Peter Jennings. In silence we have the chance to listen for our own voices, says Dr. Davis. We make choices based on what we really want and not on what others expect.

Trappist monks, Quakers, and spiritual practitioners of many other paths describe the ultimate reward of silence as a deep sense of inner peace that leads to a feeling of connection with God, nature, and all beings. "Silence leads us to listen very carefully," explains Peggy Morscheck, director of the Quaker Information Center in Philadelphia. "It

matter what's going on around us," says Dr. Rechtschaffen. Here are two quick techniques to apply whenever you notice that you've slipped from drive into overdrive.

Tune in to your body rhythms. Pay attention to your pulse or your breathing. In a study done at Tufts University in Boston, 22 middle-

---

lets us get quiet enough to hear what we Quakers call the still, small voice of God within."

This is not to suggest that you become a monk and cloister yourself for days or even hours on end. That's like the Olympics of silence. And pure silence, like that in the wilderness, a soundproof room, or an isolation tank, isn't necessary. Silence comes in a variety of shapes and sizes, from lifelong vows to weekend retreats to simply turning off the radio on your commute. Even in more modest amounts silence offers a break from external stimulation and allows you time to turn inward.

The best approach is to start with small doses, maybe 10 to 15 minutes at a time, then add more as you adapt and feel comfortable, says Dr. Kottler.

Some people have found the silence that they need just by turning off the car radio and driving in silence. Others come home to a quiet house and leave it that way, resisting the habit to turn on the stereo or pick up the phone for company. They may prepare or eat dinner in silence.

Bed is another good place to enjoy silence. One woman crawls in at night, leaves her lamp on (so she doesn't snooze), and sits for 10 to 15 minutes thinking about her day. Another sets her alarm 20 minutes early to luxuriate in early-morning serenity.

Once comfortable with short spells, you may wish to advance to a silent retreat. One of the rules at many silent retreats is no communication of any kind—including books, radios, newspapers, conversations, and eye contact. The point of removing outer stimuli is to force a turning inward. "At first, being cut off was terrifying," admits one 25-year-old woman who went on a five-day Jesuit silent retreat designed to help recent college graduates focus on their goals. "In the first hour, I felt so alone that I went right to my room and ate three granola bars for comfort. But in the upcoming days of silence, I discovered coping mechanisms that I didn't know I had. I not only got to know myself better but gained a powerful feeling of self-reliance."

age women who were highly anxious spent 10 minutes a day simply paying attention to their heart rates using wireless monitors. At the end of 12 weeks, their anxiety levels had dropped to normal.

Lead researcher James Rippe, M.D., wasn't particularly surprised by that drop. "Focusing on natural body rhythms can be very soothing," he says, because it makes the mind focus on something that's happening right now instead of letting the mind race off and worry about future concerns.

You don't have to have a heart monitor to tune in to your rhythms. A natural body rhythm that's easier to follow than your heartbeat is your breath. To learn how to focus on it, sit in a quiet place and let your eyes close. Observe yourself inhaling and exhaling. Don't try to slow your breath or make it deeper; just let it be natural. Focus on the sensation of breath as it passes through your nostrils or the back of your throat, as it lifts your belly. Practice this anywhere from 2 to 20 minutes every day. Once you get the hang of it, you can practice "watching your breath" for shorter periods anytime, anywhere. Even though you shouldn't try to slow your breath or heart rate during this exercise, it may happen naturally and produce an even more relaxing rhythm.

Take a deep breath. If you're rushing around at high speed, it's likely that your breath is racing, too. The body's reason for faster breathing is to provide more oxygen so that it can better fight or flee.

But if you shift that fast-paced breathing pattern into a long "ahhh," you mentally slow down, says Dr. Rechtschaffen. Sometimes, you can start to downshift your breathing by letting out a deep sighlike exhale. A more practiced way to go about slowing your breathing is to draw the breath as deep down in your belly as possible. The extra time that it takes to draw a deep breath as opposed to a shallow one may set your breathing back on a normal track. To make sure that you are breathing deeply enough, place your hands on your abdomen, just below your belly button. As you begin to inhale a breath slowly, feel your belly expand. If it doesn't move, you're not drawing the breath deeply enough. Lie on your back and practice on the floor, where it's easier to relax and breathe deeper.

Rehearse the Rhythms

Beyond these techniques that can be called on at any time of the day, it's a good idea to take regular forays into activities that intentionally nurture a slower rhythm.

Go wild. Seek the rhythm of nature. Outdoors, our senses have the chance to tune in to the world working at its own pace, without any artificially induced rushing (alarm clocks and beepers, to name just a couple). We see tree branches swaying gently in the wind and water meandering down its path. We watch the seasons come and go, but not overnight. Change in nature happens progressively.

For many people the biggest challenge in getting in sync with these rhythms is allowing that sync to happen rather than forcing it. When you stroll through the woods, sit along the seashore, or hang out among your daisies, don't "do" anything—just walk or sit and soak up the sights and sounds. Let them draw you into a slower pace.

Relax with a group activity. Participating in activities—with at least one other person—that require rhythmic movement, such as quilting, paddling a canoe, or sharing a meal and conversation, naturally shifts us out of a gear that's too high. "Because ordinary human social interaction is rhythmic, it seems that humans prefer smooth patterns with continuity and regularity," says Dr. Erickson. "Random, erratic patterns make us feel jumpy and on edge. Repetitive motion brings feelings of safety and satisfaction and allows us to slow down and relax."

Slow down, you're going too fast. Most of the time, transportation is something that we endure in order to get where we're going. Fixed on the destination—say, the video store—we want the trip to go fast. It's not practical in every case, but every now and then, it can be valuable to take a slower route. Walk, don't drive. Take a train instead of a plane. Drive in the right-hand lane. Traveling more leisurely lets you get immersed in enjoying the trip for its own sake (as opposed to letting your mind race ahead to what's coming next).

Move to a steady beat. Whether it's rocking or walking, humans attune quickly to slow, steady beats. "Babies love to be rocked because the tempo is slow, smooth, and consistent," says Dr. Erickson. Rocking chairs, porch swings, and hammocks offer time out from a hectic life by slowing a rapid pace. Even a stroll can be relaxing, if the strides are smooth and consistent.

The Upside of Downshifting

"Slowing down is powerful because it allows us to be more fully attentive in any given moment," says Dr. Rechtschaffen. "And when you're fully focused on the task at hand, you're able to enjoy it more and give it

(continued on page 230)

Stretch for Stress Relief

So you're stressed-out, and right now, you can't chill in a hot tub or take a 10-minute tropical vacation. And you think that your only short-term options are (1) grinning and bearing it or (2) prolonged grinning and bearing it. What do you do?

Well, you can stretch. "Stress makes muscles tense up, and stretching helps them relax," says Michael McKee, Ph.D., head of the section of health psychology at the Cleveland Clinic Foundation. "That makes you feel calmer, signaling to your brain that you're safe and everything is okay."

Stretching also helps you breathe deeper, he says, another cracker-jack method for switching off the body's emergency arousal system.

You may find that the particular stretch suggested below works on your mind as well, helping you focus your attention on your body and screen out mental distractions.

"When you narrow down your concentration and do it passively, you induce the relaxation response, which calms you," Dr. McKee says. "And when you're calm, you perform any task more efficiently."

The important thing while in this stretch, says John Friend, certified Iyengar yoga instructor and creator of the video *Yoga: Alignment and Form*, is not to strain or push.

Become aware of your right and left sides and your front and back, and try to balance the weight of all these. "Finding balance on the outside can help you feel more emotionally calm and balanced within," Friend says.

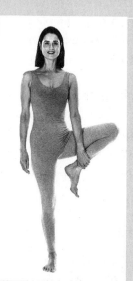

Getting into Position

Start by standing tall, feet parallel and bare, arms at your sides. Find a fixed object in front of you and softly gaze at it. Shift your weight onto your right foot. Bending your left knee, slide your left foot as high on your inner right leg as you can. Use your left hand to bring up that foot as high as possible—bending over as far as necessary to catch the left ankle. It's fine if your left foot comes only as high as your right knee or calf. You can even have the raised foot at ankle height, with your toes resting on the floor for balance, with your knee pointing out to the side. If you can't balance independently, stand with your back several inches from a wall and lean back for support as needed.

Helpful hints: Your foot will stick better if your legs are bare. To balance, plant your standing leg firmly, as if it were a tree trunk—pressing down into the floor with all four corners of your foot. If you can't balance independently, stand with your back several inches from a wall and lean back for support as needed.

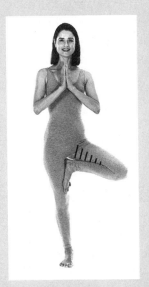

Being There

Once your foot is secure, bring your palms together at your chest. Breathe evenly and balance for up to 30 seconds. On an exhalation, gracefully lower your arms and bent leg. Repeat on the other side.

Helpful hint: Don't let your body sag. Keep your leg muscles strongly lifting, your hips firm, and your torso stretching upward.

For More Challenge:

Extend your arms out to the sides, turn the palms of your hands up, and stretch them overhead

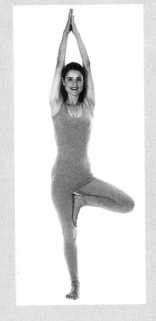

until your palms meet. (Keep your arms parallel if your palms don't reach.) Straighten your elbows and stretch the entire length of your sides, with your arms and fingers up.

Caution: *Do not take your arms overhead if you have rotator cuff injuries, cardiac problems, or high blood pressure (even if medication you take controls it).*

your best." Feeling unstressed and in sync not only may help you think more clearly but it also helps you safeguard your health. Every moment your mind is barreling into the future pulls you out of your natural rhythms and starts to activate the fight-or-flight response—the release of hormones that make your heart speed up, your muscles tighten, and your breath quicken. Some mind-body researchers believe that if this reaction happens repeatedly over time, it may lead to major health problems, including heart disease, stomach upset, insomnia, low immunity, and more.

As you first begin to participate in more leisurely activities, expect some internal resistance. When hyper is habit, slowing down can initially make us feel bored, lazy, and guilty and cause other undesirable reactions. But regular practice can help you recover a joyful sense of tranquillity and equanimity that you'll learn to call up at any time when you feel harried.

"Once you learn to shift your own internal rhythm at will, it gets easier to function in a hectic world," says Dr. Rechtschaffen. "That gives you a wonderful sense of control over your life."

Women's Health

Eating well, experts say, is the key to staying breast cancer–free. Here's how to revise all your meals to achieve potential protection.

For catching breast cancer in its earliest stages, there are mammograms plus breast self-exams plus physician exams. That's the gold standard, bar none.

But wouldn't you love a gold standard for catching breast cancer before it ever gets started? The fact is, we may already have one. According to many experts, it's diet that holds the secret to preventing this disease that women fear most.

Consider some evidence. In the United States, breast cancer rates are four to seven times higher than in Asia. But when Asian women move to the United States, their breast cancer risk doubles in 10 years and reach our rates in several generations, says nutritional epidemiologist Regina Ziegler, Ph.D., of the National Cancer Institute in Bethesda, Maryland.

What changes? "Their diets and other lifestyle factors," Dr. Ziegler says. They start eating more calories, fats, and meats and stop eating as many vegetables, fruits, grains, and soy as they did in Asia. Weight goes up and levels of exercise decrease. Which particular changes promote breast cancer? Perhaps one...perhaps all—something that future studies should tell.

And don't let news reports about the discovery of breast cancer genes fool you, either. Dr. Ziegler says that genetics and family history may explain only a small fraction of breast cancer; the majority of cases are due to something in our daily environment—with diet a likely player.

The only hitch is that more research is needed to arrive at a final verdict on the perfect diet to fight breast cancer. But there's absolutely no reason for women to wait for that day to arrive, because right now, we already know or suspect plenty about the best anti–breast cancer diet. Here are some suggestions about ways to steer your menus in a breast-protection direction.

Cut the Calories

Study after study confirms that after menopause, the more overweight the woman, the higher her risk of breast cancer. And the risk from being overweight may start in our forties, according to a study of Asian-American women from Dr. Ziegler. Women in their fifties who gained 11 or more pounds within the previous 10 years had twice the risk of developing breast cancer compared with women with no weight change. But now the silver lining: In the same study losing weight in the previous decade was associated with a 30 percent decrease in breast cancer risk. Apparently, it's never too late to slim down. If you follow the guidelines to prevent breast cancer that are outlined in this chapter, you should automatically find yourself losing excess pounds.

But why should weight loss be a factor in preventing breast cancer?

Though we're far from knowing exactly the many ways that diet affects breasts, one intriguing link turns up again and again. That link is the hormone estrogen.

Breast cancer experts believe that a lifetime of bombardment by our body's own estrogen can trigger breast tissue to become cancerous. Some scientists have suggested that certain foods may protect us from estrogen bombardment—sometimes because the foods actually contain weaker, less harmful forms of estrogen. On the other hand, weighing too much—having excess body fat—may be especially risky because fat is one of the body's estrogen factories. After menopause, when estrogen production by the ovaries takes a nosedive, fat tissue can still keep churning out estrogen.

Fruit and Veg Out

Aim for a minimum of five servings of vegetables and fruits every day. And if you can eat even more, that's a healthy plus.

Many studies now show that women who eat lots of fruits and veg-

Can You Walk Away from Breast Cancer?

Look on your closet floor. Behind the socks that you thought you'd lost and next to the shirts that slipped off the hanger, you might find your best protection against breast cancer. Don those sneakers that have been on the closet floor for so long and you might be able to outrun the breast cancer statistics. Compelling research suggests that if every woman gave her workout shoes a run (or walk) for their money, the number of breast cancer cases—which now tops 182,000 per year—could be reduced by as much as a third.

Previously, scientists have linked exercise to lower breast cancer risk. And a study of more than 5,000 women in Italy offers more evidence that easy-to-get moderate exercise—even moving around on the job—may be enough to take some of the sting out of the statistics.

In this study women in their thirties who had active jobs (moving around for the whole day) had almost half the breast cancer risk as the least active women. Take heart if you're a desk jockey. Thirty-something women who did more than sit around in their off hours also saw breast cancer risk tumble—those active more than 7 hours a week had a 24 percent lower breast cancer risk than did women who were active fewer than 2 hours a week, according to studies.

As in previous studies, younger, more active women saw the biggest benefits from on-the-job activity. Women in their fifties who had active occupations also saw a 38 percent reduction in risk. Off-the-job

etables are less likely to get breast cancer. In one study published in the *Journal of the National Cancer Institute,* women in New York State who ate more than five servings of vegetables daily had half the risk of breast cancer of women who ate fewer than three servings.

The same study showed that a rainbow of produce had a protective effect: tomatoes, spinach, greens, corn, carrots, summer squash, cucumbers, melons, berries, apples, pears, raisins, lemons, and limes. In a word, variety. On the other hand, diet supplements in pill form, such as vitamins C and E and folic acid, offered no protection.

What's at work here? "We used to think that it was a particular mineral or vitamin or antioxidant," says John Pierce, Ph.D., head of cancer

physical activity held its protection nearly steady in women in their fifties, though after menopause, activity's effect on breast cancer risk wasn't as strong.

"Before menopause, exercise may reduce the exposure of women's breast cells to hormones," says Leslie Bernstein, Ph.D., pioneer of breast cancer/exercise research at the University of Southern California School of Medicine in Los Angeles. Especially in young women, moderate exercise is believed to alter the menstrual cycle so that there is less estrogen and progesterone roaming around in their bodies offering a warm bed to cancers that feel like taking up residence.

This doesn't let postmenopausal women off the hook. "Exercise done after menopause will have a small effect," says Dr. Bernstein. "It's likely to have an effect through the reduction of body fat, resulting in lower hormonal exposure of breast cells to estrogens that are produced by the action of an enzyme in body fat on an adrenal hormone."

That women might be able to keep cancer risk from sneaking up by putting their sneakers on is some of the best breast news so far. It means that there's a promise that scientists' hard work will soon pay off. Plus, exercise isn't the only thing that you can do to keep risk down. Staying at a sensible weight and eating low-fat foods and maybe even foods full of soy may be smart. "But since it has so many health benefits," says Dr. Bernstein, "a woman would be negligent if she did not include a regular exercise program (30 to 40 minutes a day) as part of her lifestyle."

Self-Serving

Ever wonder what nutritionists mean when they say "one serving?" Here are the portions that they're talking about.

One Serving of Veggies and Fruits Is Equal to:

1 cup raw leafy vegetables

$\frac{1}{2}$ cup other vegetables (cooked or chopped raw)

$\frac{3}{4}$ cup vegetable or fruit juice

1 medium apple, banana, or orange

$\frac{1}{2}$ cup fruit (chopped, cooked, frozen, or canned)

2 tablespoons dried fruit

prevention at the University of San Diego Cancer Center. "Now we know that it's more complex. In effect, a variety of produce works like a soup filled with weak anti-carcinogens. You need to drink the whole soup for maximum effect."

Dr. Pierce is studying the power of veggies and fruits to fight recurrence of cancer in 3,000 women who have had breast cancer. The Women's Healthy Eating and Living (WHEL) trial will test a diet that's ultrahigh in veggies, fruits, and fiber and ultralow in fat.

But the diet is already getting a trial run from Cyndi Thomson, a registered dietitian in Arizona, who has served as a co-site director for the WHEL study. Thomson made a commitment to eat the same diet as the women in the study, including loads of vegetables and fruits. And she made that commitment even though her schedule—as with many other people—allows little time for special preparations. Working on a job and a Ph.D., with two young sons and a husband to feed, Thomson never has much time to spend in the kitchen.

To make "ultra" eating possible, Thomson developed a number of super-easy strategies to make sure that her family gets all the veggies and fruits that the diet calls for. In the first year after Thomson changed her diet, her husband lost 15 excess pounds (she didn't lose because she was already trim). Thomson didn't catch one cold. And her two young sons began snacking on fruit instead of the usual junk food. Here are Thomson's tips to help you get feasts from the fruit of the Earth.

Make it convenient. Thomson stocks both her office and car with fruits and vegetables, keeping a mini-cooler in the car. On her last out-of-town trip, she ordered a fruit basket from the hotel. "It was $22, but I got about 25 pieces of fruit, enough to last my whole trip."

Keep it fresh. Thomson shops for most groceries once a week, but she makes sure that produce is fresh by restocking midweek.

Send in the salsa. "I push a lot of salsa—there are so many great varieties in stores," Thomson says. "But I doctor them up with my own vegetables and fruits—chopped cucumber, broccoli, or kiwi, usually."

Dine out creatively. "When you're eating out, you have to stick up for yourself and ask for what you want," Thomson says. At a conference lunch serving lasagna, a side vegetable, and a salad, she skipped the lasagna and had two sides of veggies and a salad instead.

Make some for the fridge. "We always have cut-up vegetables in the fridge," Thomson says. "Every time I'm cutting up vegetables anyway, for a meal or something, I cut up a few more for the fridge."

Make it visible. "I have a well-stocked fruit basket on the table and see-through drawers in the fridge so that I always know what's in there," Thomson says.

Sneak 'em in. "I add shredded carrots or chopped-up zucchini to store-bought spaghetti sauce," says Thomson. "I still buy packaged low-sodium rice and pasta mixes, but now I throw in vegetables or legumes. We make fajitas, but instead of using mostly meat or chicken, ours are mostly grilled green and sweet red peppers and onions."

Choose the best. Though all veggies and fruits are superstars, some deserve top billing. Here are the ones to select for special protection.

- Leafy greens like spinach, yellow vegetables like squash, and orange veggies like carrots are high in beta-carotene, which has protective effects.
- Cabbage and its relatives—broccoli, cauliflower, brussels sprouts, and kale—have a compound called indole-3-carbinol, or I3C, that steps up the body's production of a weaker, less carcinogenic form of estrogen. This veggie clan also has sulforaphane, a compound that encourages the body's own breast cancer–fighting enzymes.
- Preliminary studies in animals and test tubes indicate that compounds in the juices of oranges, grapefruit, and tangerines can help stop breast cancer cell growth, according to the journal *Nutrition and Cancer*.

Fill Up on Fiber

Doctors recommend that you get 30 grams of fiber daily from a variety of sources, including vegetables and fruits, whole grains, and dried beans.

In Finland, for instance, where women consume 30 grams of fiber daily (compared with our 14 grams), the rate of breast cancer is only half that of women's in the United States.

"We have quite strong evidence showing that fiber is protective," says David Rose, M.D., of the American Health Foundation. Dr. Rose showed in a study that 30 grams of fiber a day—half from food and half from added wheat bran—dropped women's estrogen levels by 20 percent. Another reason that fiber may help is that lots of antioxidants and other protective compounds are found in high-fiber foods.

The Gram Total of Fiber

To help you make sure that you're getting your 30 grams of fiber each day, here's a list of some good fiber sources to choose from.

5 grams of fiber each

$\frac{1}{2}$ cup cooked dried beans, peas, or lentils

1 serving of a high-fiber wheat-bran cereal*

2 grams of fiber each

1 serving of a fruit or vegetable (not counting juice)**

1 slice whole-wheat bread

$\frac{1}{2}$ cup whole-wheat pasta

$\frac{1}{2}$ whole-wheat bagel

1 slice rye crisp bread

1 gram of fiber

1 serving of a refined grain food*

*See package for serving size.
**See "Self-Serving" on page 234 for serving sizes.

You'll reach 30 grams of fiber with five servings of fruits and vegetables, five servings of whole grains, one serving of a high-fiber wheat-bran cereal, and one serving of dried beans. Always pick whole-wheat products when you can and make white bread or white pasta the exception rather than the rule.

Degrease

Keep fat to 20 percent of total calories maximum. That's the level currently being tested to prevent breast cancer in the giant Women's Health Initiative study sponsored by the National Institutes of Health in Bethesda, Maryland.

Peter Greenwald, M.D., director of cancer prevention at the National Cancer Institute, is just one of many researchers who has concluded that a low-fat diet is helpful in preventing breast cancer. He points to research showing that there are lower rates of breast cancer in countries

Your 20 Percent Fat Budget

Although the link between dietary fat and breast cancer is unclear, some researchers are convinced that eating a diet that includes no more than 20 percent of calories from fat can reduce a woman's risk of developing the disease.

To figure fat-gram budgets based on 20 percent of calories, multiply your average daily calorie intake by 0.20, then divided by 9 (since each fat gram contains 9 calories). Or you can use this handy chart. Just find the approximate number of calories that you eat in a day. Then look to see how many grams of fat should be your maximum intake to keep your daily fat calories at 20 percent.

Calories	Fat (g.)
1,200	27
1,400	31
1,600	36
1,800	40
2,000	44
2,200	49

around the world where less fat is eaten. Even within the same country, like Japan, breast cancer rises as Japanese women eat a larger percentage of calories from fat. Your safest bet, says Dr. Greenwald, is to go low-fat (also, get some exercise and keep your calories in check).

Find your fat-gram maximum, based on average calories that you eat in a day, in "Your 20 Percent Fat Budget" on page 237. Then, add up the grams of fat that you eat throughout the day. Almost all packaged foods give grams of fat per serving on their labels. For most restaurant meals you'll have to estimate.

Curb the Cocktails

Have no more than two to three alcohol-containing drinks in one week, research suggests, and you'll cut your risk of breast cancer.

A major review of the alcohol–and–breast cancer connection, published in *Cancer Causes and Control*, found that, on average, women having one drink a day had an 11 percent higher risk of breast cancer. But there's a complication here in what's best for our overall health, since one drink a day seems to protect us from heart attacks, acknowledges Walter Willett, M.D., head of nutrition at the Harvard School of Public Health.

What to do? "If you don't have risk factors for heart disease, then the benefit from alcohol is small and outweighed by the higher risk of breast cancer," Dr. Willet says.

The risk is minimal if you stay at two to three drinks per week, according to Dr. Willet. (One drink is considered to be a 5-ounce glass of wine, a 12-ounce beer, or a drink made with 1½ ounces of 80-proof distilled spirits.) "So if you enjoy wine, for example, have it infrequently and get a very good bottle," he suggests.

Stick with Soy

Get a daily intake of soy foods with 30 to 50 milligrams of isoflavones, and you'll enhance your body's ability to fend off breast cancer.

"In Asian countries, where soy is a staple, there's a marked lowering of breast cancer," notes soy expert Kenneth Setchell, Ph.D., of the University of Cincinnati College of Medicine. Dr. Setchell is convinced that the compounds in soy called isoflavones make the difference. The average Asian consumes an estimated 50 or more milligrams of isoflavones in soy foods daily. Isoflavones act like weak estrogens once inside the body. In theory, they prevent breast cancer by occupying landing sites on breast cells and blocking out stronger, cancer-promoting human estrogen. Not all soy foods have isoflavones; soy sauce and soybean oil actually have very little. But other soy products and sources can give you the cancer-fighting isoflavones that you need.

For starters, try soy milk in puddings or on cereal, blend tofu in fruit smoothies, or make a soy butter and jelly sandwich. One-quarter cup of roasted soy nuts has about 60 milligrams of isoflavones. Other good sources are ½ cup of tempeh or tofu—both have about 35 milligrams. A 1-cup serving of regular soy milk has about 30 milligrams, and 1 cup of low-fat soy milk contains about 20 milligrams of isoflavones.

Feast on Flaxseed

In animal studies flaxseed helps keep breast cancer from starting and slows the growth of tumors already under way. Researchers give the credit to a compound most plentiful in flaxseed—something called lignan precursors. In the body these compounds convert to weak estrogens that may behave like soy's isoflavones. Your goal, say researchers, should be about one serving of flaxseed (up to 25 grams) per day. To get this amount, sprinkle 2 heaping tablespoons of ground flaxseed on cereal or in juice.

Get into Garlic

Eat one-half to one clove of garlic several times a week, doctors say, and you'll be on the track to cutting your risk.

Researchers at Memorial Sloan-Kettering Cancer Center in New York City have shown in test tube studies that four of garlic's pungent compounds stop human breast cells from becoming cancerous. They also appear to change estrogens to less cancer-promoting forms.

Researchers' consensus is that garlic probably has benefits whether it's eaten raw or cooked, so have it either way.

Careful with Meat—And Watch How You Cook It

A study from Uruguay, South America, where people eat lots of meat, found that women who ate the most meat had over three times the risk of breast cancer as those eating the least. Those eating the most red meat had four times the risk. But fried meat was the absolute worst. The top consumers had five times the risk of breast cancer, according to the *International Journal of Cancer.*

This doesn't surprise Barbara Pence, Ph.D., of Texas Tech University Health Sciences Center in Lubbock. Her own research has shown that frying and broiling, especially to well-done, produce cancer-causing substances—heterocyclic amines—even in poultry and fish.

To cook meat without cooking up heterocyclic amines, try braising, slow roasting, or microwaving. Will grilling veggie or soy burgers produce heterocyclic amines? Probably not, says Dr. Pence, because proteins in non-animal–source burgers are different.

Catch Some Fish Oil

Try for a serving of high omega-3 fish three times a week. Diets high in fish oils (omega-3 fatty acids) have been shown to slow the growth and spread of breast cancer tumors in animals. Indirect evidence links omega-3 fatty acids to human breast cancer: In a study of women having breast cancer surgery, a higher amount of alpha-linolenic acid in fat tissue around tumors was associated with a decreased spread of cancer. The link? Alpha-linolenic acid is a plant fatty acid that the body converts to the same omega-3 fatty acids found in fish oils. By the way, flaxseed is high in alpha-linolenic acid, another way that it may protect your breasts.

For lots of omega-3's, count on any canned or fresh salmon (not smoked salmon or lox) and canned white (albacore) tuna.

part

4

Timely Paths to Natural Health

An Overview of the Best New

Programs, Plans, and Ideas

in Natural Healing

Super Foods

You can count on this potent quintet to deliver cheap and delectable protection against disease and infection.

Imagine that you are stranded on an uninhabited island. Suddenly, you spy a crate labeled "perishable" washed up on the beach. As you dash toward it, your mind races—Steak? Ice cream? Beer? But if you were fortunate, it would contain a bounty of the following fruits and vegetables—all of them nutritional powerhouses capable of boosting your body's natural immunity. Here's a closer look.

Super Food #1: Asparagus

A ½-cup serving of asparagus packs more than double the total dietary fiber of red cabbage and 10 times that of one passion fruit. Plus, asparagus has more folic acid than three oranges. It also contains a splash of vitamin C, a burst of iron, a significant show of B vitamins, and only 22 fat-free calories.

Selecting and Storing

- Look for firm, green stalks with deep green or purplish tips tightly closed and compact. Size is not a marker of quality; thin or thick, the same freshness rules apply.
- Avoid wet spears and those with an odor and excessively sandy spears (sand lodges in tips and can be difficult to wash out).
- Trim 1 inch from the bottoms. Stand it upright in 1 inch of water and refrigerate. Or, wrap the bottoms in damp paper towels and store in the crisper for up to three days.
- Before cooking, snap off woody bottoms; they'll break above the stalk's tough part.

Enjoying

Less is more. The less you do, the better. Simply steam asparagus in a narrow pot in 1 inch of water (add a lemon slice or garlic clove) for 5 minutes. Drain and drizzle with lemon juice or orange juice. Or cool, then serve it with a light vinaigrette.

Save the stems. Set aside the stems and puree them for sauces or soups.

Break away from tradition. Scramble up ¾ cup nonfat egg substitute with chopped scallions, top with 2 or 3 stalks of steamed asparagus, and encase in a flour tortilla. Sprinkle with 1 tablespoon shredded low-fat Cheddar cheese.

Super Food #2: Pomegranate

One juicy, crimson-red fruit packs more potassium than 1½ naval oranges and 150 percent more dietary fiber than a cup of brown rice. Pomegranate also delivers a helpful boost of vitamin C, most of the B vitamins, copper, pantothenic acid, magnesium, and phosphorus ... with less than 1 gram of fat and only 105 calories. And it's delightfully messy.

Selecting and Storing

- A pomegranate is about as big as a large orange, and the larger it is, the sweeter. Look for rich, dark red, leathery skin that is blemish-free. If powdery clouds puff from the fruit's crown when pressed, move on (it's too dry).
- Refrigerate whole fruit for up to three months. Seeds can be packed tightly in an airtight container and frozen for just as long.

Enjoying

Get to know it. Minimalists can simply cut open and scoop out the scarlet, juicy-crisp capsulelike seeds. Or roll the whole fruit on a hard surface to break the pulpy pockets, take a small bite, and suck the unusually sweet yet tart nectar. But try not to get any on you—it stains.

Then play around. That same rich cranberry-red color makes this fruit a holiday natural. Garnish a Thanksgiving or Christmas bird; swirl the capsules in punch or pumpkin soup; put the crowning touch on ices and ice creams; or mix the pulpy capsules with nonfat cream cheese, form into sweet-tart little balls, and roll in a dusting of ground walnuts.

Make jelly. Place pomegranate's fleshy seeds over low heat until the juice flows freely. Strain without pressure (allow to drip all night if necessary), then follow a basic apple-jelly recipe.

Use it as a condiment. Boil down the juice to a thick syrup. Use it in drinks, sorbets, and marinades or as a sauce—it's especially great brushed over baked apples, poached pears, or kibbeh patties (a Middle Eastern delicacy of seasoned ground lamb) before grilling.

Add a splash of color. Give your salad greens a fabulous crimson touch: Add pureed pomegranate to French dressing; then toss in some whole seeds.

Super Food #3: Prunes

Six large, deep purple dried plums serve up five times the fiber of ½ cup of apple slices—skins on—with four times the magnesium found in a slice of oat-bran bread. Prunes also contain more iron than 3 ounces of a lean cut of eye-of-round beef. Plus, they yield a substantial amount of potassium and B vitamins and contain a special compound called dihydroxyphenyl isatin—a natural laxative. That six-prune serving contains less than ½ gram of fat and only 200 calories. So snack away.

Selecting and Storing

- Packaging is critical in purchasing prunes. Be sure that they're tightly sealed, ensuring moistness and cleanliness. Vacuum-packed are the best—those prunes are most moist.
- Buy small or large; size has no relation to flavor or quality. And pitting has only to do with cost: Pitted prunes are more expensive. But pits are easily removed through a small knife slit.
- To store, reseal the package tightly or transfer the prunes to an airtight container. Keep in a cool, dry place or refrigerate for up to six months.

Enjoying

Plump them up. Prunes are a superb chew right out of the package. But if you prefer them soft and plump, you can prepare them quickly on the stove. In a saucepan, combine any amount of prunes with an equal amount of orange juice or apple juice and flavor with cinnamon, cloves, nutmeg, citrus zest, and vanilla extract (or a few seeds from a bean). Bring to a boil over medium heat.

Bake a compote. You can make a delicious compote for dessert. Just add dried or fresh apricots, pears, cherries, pineapple, and some curry powder to the boiled mixture that you prepare on the stove. After you let the mixture cool, place the plump prunes in a baking dish and heat for 30 minutes. Serve with a dollop of nonfat vanilla yogurt or cascade over angel-food cake.

Make mousse. In a high-speed blender or food processor, combine 20 pitted prunes that have been softened by boiling. Add 1 envelope dissolved gelatin, ¾ cup nonfat ricotta cheese, ¾ cup skim milk, 1 teaspoon vanilla extract, and ¼ teaspoon nutmeg. Pour into molds that have been lightly coated with nonstick spray and refrigerate until firm.

Substitute for fat. Prunes can replace fat in baked goods. Puree 1⅓ cups prunes with 6 tablespoons hot water and process in a blender or food processor until smooth (or simply buy a jar of prune butter, or lekvar). Use in cakes, muffins, and brownies in measurements equal to oil or butter.

Super Food #4: Tofu

A mere ½ cup of this mild-tasting, cheeselike product (when it's been prepared with calcium sulfate) delivers nearly twice as much calcium as an equal amount of regular cottage cheese or as much as 1 ounce of part-skim mozzarella cheese. Tofu serves up as much iron as a 3-ounce serving of roasted eye of round and twice as much protein as a hot dog. Plus, it yields a healthy boost of isoflavones, those likely foes of breast and prostate cancer as well as osteoporosis. Yet it only has only 106 calories.(Check labels for calcium amounts; even products made with calcium sulfate have varying levels.)

Selecting and Storing

- Tofu is sold in four textures: *Soft* and *silken* have a custardlike texture, and they're a natural in dips, dressings, custards, cheesecakes, and puddings. *Firm,* with its medium-dense texture, holds its shape admirably when cut up in salads, casseroles, barbecues, and soups. *Extra-firm* is just that—really firm. Use this style for stir-frying or crumbling or just slice it for a sandwich in place of cheese.
- Use tofu straight from the box or package. No cooking is necessary. Some tofu products, sterilized through a modern process called aseptic pasteurization, can be stored unopened at room temperature for up to 10 months. You won't find these products in the dairy case. Instead, look for these boxes on regular supermarket shelves. Once opened, refrigerate and use the tofu within two days. Fresh tofu, packaged as cakes floating in water, should be re-

frigerated, and the water should be changed daily. Be sure to adhere to sell-by dates when purchasing. Don't buy a bloated container, and toss out tofu with a strong odor.

Enjoying

Dunk it. Tofu has a memory like a steel trap, soaking up and remembering any flavor that it comes in contact with (its blandness is a huge bonus in that department—there are no conflicting tastes). Cut chunks into soups, stews, chili, or marinara sauce.

Drink it. In a blender, combine ½ cup fresh red raspberries, ½ cup nonfat plain yogurt, ½ cup soft or silken tofu, ½ cup skim milk, and a dash of vanilla extract. Sweeten with honey to taste.

Spread it. Blend ½ pound soft tofu with ¼ cup confectioners' sugar, 1 tablespoon margarine, 1 teaspoon vanilla extract, and ½ teaspoon coconut extract. Spread over the crown of an angel-food cake and sprinkle with toasted coconut.

Flip it. Make tofu burgers. In a large bowl, mash 1 pound extra-firm tofu with ½ cup cooked rice, ½ cup dry bread crumbs, ½ cup scallions, 1 tablespoon chicken-flavor seasoning, ¼ cup grated carrots, ¼ cup grated low-fat Cheddar cheese, and 1 tablespoon low-sodium soy sauce. Form into patties and sauté in a skillet till golden.

Super Food #5: Pumpkin

Pumpkin has carved out a special niche among the super foods. Just 1 cup of cooked, pureed pumpkin packs more beta-carotene than an equal amount of cantaloupe or cooked dried apricots. It surpasses broccoli and corn in dietary fiber and contains more iron than one 3½-ounce serving of extra-lean ground beef. Pumpkin also has twice as much magnesium as kale and offers a substantial boost of vitamin C plus a smidgen of niacin, riboflavin, copper, and vitamin B_6. All this with less than 1 gram of fat and only 83 calories.

Selecting and Storing

- Pass on the jack-o'-lantern variety; it's too tough and stringy. For cooking always choose a sugar-pie pumpkin—a smaller, sweeter variety with a finer flesh.
- Select a pumpkin with no cracks or soft spots, and make sure it has a rounded, dry stem. If the stem is blackened or moist, move on.

- Store in a cool, dry place, uncut, for up to one month. If cut, wrap tightly and refrigerate for up to one week.
- Buy canned. It's an excellent alternative; it's just as pure, equally nutritious, and so quick and easy.

Enjoying

Simplify. Here's the easiest way to prepare fresh pumpkin: Rinse the pumpkin, cut it in half, and scoop out the seeds and stringy fibers. Place the pumpkin, cut side down, in a baking dish with ¼ inch of water. Bake at 350°F for about 45 minutes, then remove from the oven. When cool, scoop out the soft flesh and drain in a colander. Puree in a food processor, then drain again thoroughly. Use immediately or freeze for up to nine months in 1-cup containers for later use.

Slim your pumpkin. Spice up the autumn air with your favorite pumpkin recipes, but reduce the fat: For pumpkin pie, use evaporated skim milk instead of cream, and egg substitute instead of eggs. Buy a low-fat graham-cracker crust. For pumpkin bread, replace the oil with half as much prune puree and use egg substitute. Or, brew a warm, cozy pumpkin soup using evaporated skim milk instead of heavy cream.

Be innovative. Slather canned or fresh pumpkin puree mixed with molasses (to taste) on a multigrain, nonfat toasted waffle for a nutritious breakfast, lunch, or snack.

Everyday Herbal Meals That Heal

Using herbs in your favorite foods not only arouses the taste buds but also may cure what ails you. Here's how to cook with these fabulous natural healers.

No kitchen is really complete without herbs. They are absolutely essential for bringing out the best flavors in low-fat, low-salt recipes.

They can even be an unexpected source of vitamins and minerals.

Fresh parsley, for example, contains vitamins A and C, calcium, iron, and potassium. And other herbs are also surprisingly decent sources of various nutrients.

But the real power of herbs is their knack for transforming ordinary dishes into medicinal marvels—as in the recipes that follow, created by Judith Benn Hurley, author of *The Good Herb: Remedies and Recipes from Nature.*

In virtually every country around the world, herbal foods are used in one form or another to prevent or heal diseases like hay fever, prostate problems, asthma, headaches, menopause, fatigue, and stress. In India, for example, vegetables like cauliflower and cabbage are cooked in mustard seed to prevent digestive troubles. In Russia, dill seed is steeped in cooking oil, then massaged into the hands to strengthen nails and soften cuticles. In Zimbabwe, basil tea is a dandruff remedy.

Granted, most people don't use herbs in large enough quantities to take advantage of this bonus. But you can look for ways to significantly increase your use of herbs—especially fresh ones. If herb cookery is new to you, start with modest amounts. As you come to enjoy these bold flavors, be more generous. Throw handfuls of parsley, basil, dill, or coriander, for instance, into salads, stir-fries, quiches, and pasta dishes.

Make herbs an important part of your repertoire, and they'll reward you beyond measure. To get you started, here are some healing herbal dishes for breakfast, lunch, and dinner.

Best Blends

Mix up these all-purpose dried-herb combinations and keep them handy for quick meals. Pulverize the herbs, place in capped shaker jars, and use while cooking and on the table. (With fresh herbs, mince only enough for immediate use.)

For poultry: equal parts basil, chervil, marjoram, parsley, and thyme

For fish: equal parts chives, celery seed, and dill

For vegetables: four parts basil, chervil, chives, marjoram, and parsley plus one part each savory and thyme

Pear and Ginger Breakfast Muffins

Some herbalists say that ginger stimulates digestion, making it a healthful addition to a morning muffin.

1½ cups bran nugget cereal

½ cup pure pear or apple juice

1 pear, coarsely grated

2 teaspoons finely grated fresh ginger

½ cup nonfat plain yogurt or soy yogurt

¼ cup all-fruit pear or apple butter

¼ cup pure maple syrup

2 large egg whites or ¼ cup Calendula Egg Substitute (see page 258)

1 tablespoon canola oil

1¼ cups unbleached all-purpose flour

2 teaspoons baking soda

1 teaspoon ground cinnamon

Preheat the oven to 400°F.

In a medium bowl, combine the cereal, pear juice or apple juice, pear, and ginger. Let the mixture soak for 10 minutes. Then stir in the yogurt, fruit, butter, syrup, egg whites or egg substitute, and oil.

In another medium bowl, combine the flour, baking soda, and cinnamon. Pour the cereal mixture into the flour mixture and use a large rubber spatula to combine. Don't overmix; about 15 strokes should be enough.

Lightly oil 12 muffin tins and divide the batter among them. Bake for 18 to 20 minutes, or until cooked through.

Makes 12 muffins

Per muffin: 136 calories, 2 g. fat

Sage and Egg Omelet

Ancient Arabic and Chinese herbalists believed that drinking sage tea enhanced mental and spiritual clarity. Modern herbalists report that sage's camphor and other volatile oils have antiseptic properties, which, when combined with the astringent action of sage's tannin, can help treat sore gums and mouth ulcers, according to Hurley. This recipe is incredibly simple, and it makes a perfect brunch for two served with a side of grilled tomatoes. The sizzled sage gives the eggs an irresistible, earthy, full aroma.

1   teaspoon olive oil

1   teaspoon sweet (unsalted) butter

7   large fresh sage leaves

3   large eggs (see note)
    Splash of water

2   tablespoons freshly grated Romano cheese or soy Parmesan cheese
    Sage or chive flowers (optional)

Heat the oil and butter in a medium nonstick skillet over medium-high heat until the butter has melted. Then use a pastry brush to distribute the fats evenly in the pan. Arrange the sage in the pan and let sizzle for about 20 seconds, or until fragrant.

Meanwhile, in a medium bowl, use a whisk to beat together the eggs and water.

Pour the egg mixture over the sage and immediately sprinkle the Parmesan on top. If necessary, rotate the pan so that the egg mixture cooks evenly. The egg mixture will set in less than 2 minutes on a gas stove and take a bit longer on an electric stove. When it's firm and no longer runny, slide the omelet onto a waiting plate, flipping half of the omelet over on itself. Serve at once, garnished with the sage or chive flowers (if using).

Note: If this is more fat than you're used to, bring it down a bit by substituting egg whites for one or two of the whole eggs. Two egg whites equals one whole egg.

Makes 2 servings

Per serving: 180 calories, 15 g. fat

Mediterranean Chicken Thighs

This French-style dish will give you good amounts of vitamin C and niacin. Both strengthen your immune system so you're less likely to come down with pesky infections. Fennel, one of the herbs in this dish, is unparalleled at relieving intestinal gas, says Hurley. By the way, although thighs aren't as lean as breast meat, you can easily pare out much of their excess fat with a knife.

4	teaspoons olive oil
1½	cups sliced onions
1	tablespoon minced garlic
1	green pepper, thinly sliced
1	sweet yellow pepper, thinly sliced
10	whole Niçoise olives or 5 pitted black olives, chopped
¼	teaspoon fennel seeds
⅛	teaspoon dried thyme
⅛	teaspoon dried rosemary
	Pinch of red-pepper flakes
1¼	pounds boneless, skinless chicken thighs, trimmed of all visible fat
2	teaspoons red-wine vinegar
⅛	teaspoon ground black pepper

Preheat the oven to 425°F.

Heat the oil in a large nonstick skillet over medium heat. Add the onions and garlic. Sauté for 4 to 5 minutes, stirring frequently, until the onions are nearly tender.

Add the green and yellow peppers. Sauté for 5 to 6 minutes, stirring frequently, until the peppers are tender. Add the olives, fennel seeds, thyme, rosemary, and red-pepper flakes. Sauté for 1 minute, stirring frequently.

Arrange the chicken in a single layer in a shallow baking dish. Drizzle with the vinegar and sprinkle with the black pepper. Spoon the vegetables over the chicken. Bake for 25 to 30 minutes, or until the chicken is cooked through and the juices run clear when you pierce the thighs with a fork.

Notes: For an accompaniment, serve the chicken with steamed asparagus and cooked pasta tossed with a splash of extra-virgin olive oil and chopped fresh basil or parsley.

To cook the vegetables in the microwave, place the oil, onions, and peppers in a 2-quart glass bowl. Cover with plastic and microwave for 3 to 5 minutes, stirring twice, until tender. Add the spices and microwave for an additional minute.

For a variation, use chicken cutlets instead of thighs. They may cook a little faster than the thighs, so check for doneness after 15 minutes. If yellow peppers are not available, use all red or a mixture of red and green.

Makes 4 servings

Per serving: 248 calories, 11.3 g. fat

Whole-Wheat Spaghetti with Sage

Sage's sharpness lifts the flavor of whole wheat.

1	tablespoon olive oil
3	cloves garlic, minced
⅓	cup vegetable stock or water
10	no-salt-added sun-dried tomato halves
¼	cup loosely packed fresh sage leaves or 2 tablespoons dried
4	cups hot cooked whole-wheat spaghetti (about 8 ounces dried)

In a small saucepan, combine the oil, garlic, stock or water, and tomatoes. Bring to a boil. Boil for about 2 minutes, or until the liquid has been reduced to about ¼ cup.

Meanwhile, toss the sage into a large serving bowl and add the spaghetti. The heat will release the aroma of the sage.

Pour the tomato mixture over the pasta, toss well, and serve warm.

Makes 4 servings

Per serving: 290 calories, 3.5 g. fat

Broccoli and Potatoes with Dill

Broccoli is a prominent and easy-to-cook member of the cruciferous family of vegetables—renowned for helping prevent certain types of cancer. And potatoes are a great source of vitamin C, vitamin B$_6$, and iron. But how can you make these health-giving vegetables more interesting? In this recipe, Hurley suggests using dill, scallions, capers, and lemon juice to give these ordinary vegetables a lift.

> **Handful of fresh dill sprigs**
> 2 **medium red potatoes(about 1 pound), cut into 1″ chunks**
> 1¼ **cups broccoli florets (about ½ pound)**
> 3 **scallions, minced**
> 2 **teaspoons minced capers**
> 3 **tablespoons fresh lemon juice**
> 1 **tablespoon olive oil**
> 1 **teaspoon minced fresh dill or ½ teaspoon dried**
> **Freshly ground black pepper**

Fill a large saucepan with water and bring to a boil over high heat. Add the dill sprigs. Place the potatoes in a steamer basket, then place over the saucepan. Steam the potatoes, covered, over the boiling water for about 5 minutes. Add the broccoli and continue steaming for about 5 more minutes, or until the vegetables are tender.

Tip the potatoes and broccoli into a large serving bowl. Add the scallions, capers, lemon juice, oil, dill, and pepper, to taste. Toss well. Serve warm as a side dish or very slightly chilled as a salad. Or use as a filling for crêpes or omelets.

Makes 4 servings

Per serving: 187 calories, 3.5 g. fat

A Potpourri of Hints

Lore about curative herbs has been passed on from generation to generation of cooks as well as herbalists. Here's a collection of herbal advice from experts who know about growing, preserving, and cooking.

- Chew on parsley sprigs after eating garlic or other strong foods to freshen your breath.
- One way to preserve the flavor of fresh herbs is to blend them with heart-healthy olive or canola oil. Among the herbs that do particularly well are basil, tarragon, rosemary, and sage. Blending in some of a crushed vitamin C tablet may help the leaves green and prevent them from losing their flavors. (Try 250 milligrams with $\frac{1}{4}$ cup oil and $\frac{1}{2}$ pound herbs.)
- Toss garlicky chive flowers or peppery nasturtium blooms into salads for color and flavor. Use other herb flowers in the same way.
- Steaming is a particularly healthy way of cooking fish and vegetables. Give them fat-free zip by laying branches of herbs across the food as it cooks. Best bets include dill, rosemary, and tarragon.
- Microwaving—which preserves vitamins in produce—also retains much more of herbs' natural flavors, so you need less. Reduce the amount of fresh herbs by a third and dried herbs by half.
- To get the most flavor when roasting meat or poultry, rub its surface well with seasonings before cooking. If preparing poultry with the skin on, loosen the skin and rub the herbs into the flesh underneath. The poultry will absorb the flavors better, and you can then discard the fatty skin before eating without losing the herb taste.
- Lighten up your tomato sandwiches. Use whole basil leaves in place of or in addition to lettuce. With their full flavor you won't need fatty mayonnaise.
- When cooking with bay leaves, be sure to remove them before serving. They never soften to the point where you can chew them properly, so you might choke on a piece if you try to eat it.
- Use mint in pea soup. It not only enriches the flavor but also counteracts the tendency of peas to produce gas.

Swordfish with Fennel

In India, fennel is chewed after meals to soothe digestion and freshen the breath. This recipe combines olive oil, wine, garlic, and fennel—all classic flavorings for fish.

- 1   teaspoon olive oil
- 2   tablespoons dry white wine
- 1–2 cloves garlic, chopped
- 1   teaspoon fennel seeds
- 1   pound swordfish steak, about ½″ thick

Preheat the broiler or prepare the grill.

Combine the oil, wine, garlic, and fennel in a mortar or spice grinder and crush to a coarse paste. Rub the paste all over the fish.

Broil or grill the fish for 3 to 4 minutes on each side, or until just cooked through. Serve warm with a salad of mustard greens.

Makes 4 servings

Per serving: 170 calories, 4.5 g. fat

Peppermint Blend Tea

Peppermint tea contains menthol, which soothes the stomach, eases digestion, and helps fend off nausea and vomiting, according to Hurley. The herb also helps relieve flu symptoms and can stop hiccups. Licorice root and peppermint give this tea sweetness without adding sugar or honey.

- 1   tablespoon + 1 teaspoon dried peppermint leaves
- 3   slices Chinese licorice root (see note)
- 2   teaspoons dried raspberry leaves
- 1   teaspoon dried lemon grass
- 1   quart boiling water

Steep the peppermint, licorice, raspberry, and lemon grass in the water, covered, for 4 minutes. Strain and discard the peppermint, raspberry, and lemon grass. Return the licorice to the tea to give it extra sweetness. Enjoy the tea hot or chilled.

Note: Chinese licorice root is available at Chinese markets and herb shops. Don't substitute European or American licorice, both of which are strong laxatives.

Makes 4 servings

Per serving: 5 calories

Traditional Kitchen Matchups

While it's true that most herbs go with most foods, there are some pairings that are especially successful.

Dried beans: cumin, sage, and thyme

Cabbage: caraway and dill

Carrots: basil, cumin, and mint

Cauliflower: dill and marjoram

Eggplant: basil, cinnamon, and oregano

Fruit: anise, ginger, and mint

Lamb: bay leaf, mint, and rosemary

Potatoes: chives, marjoram, paprika, and thyme

Spinach: dill and nutmeg

Tomatoes: basil, oregano, and tarragon

Turkey: basil, marjoram, and savory

Calendula Egg Substitute

Research hints that calendula might offer some protection against cancer since it contains beta-carotene (the plant form of vitamin A) and carotenoids. Use ¼ cup of this no-fat-added, salt- and preservative-free mixture to replace each egg in a recipe. You can't scramble it, but it's great in batters for muffins, quick breads, pancakes, waffles, and scones or as a glaze for French toast.

> 1 **cup boiling water**
>
> **Petals from 1 fresh or dried calendula blossom (about 1 tablespoon)**
>
> 1 **tablespoon flaxseed (see note)**

In a medium bowl, pour the water over the calendula petals and cover. Let steep for about 5 minutes, or until the color is a rich yellow. Strain and discard the petals.

Pour the calendula tea into a small saucepan and add the flaxseed. Bring to a boil and boil for about 3 minutes, or until the tea is reduced to about ¾ cup. Transfer the mixture to a food processor or blender and process for about 30 seconds to coarsely crush the seeds. Strain to remove most of the seeds (it's alright if some seeds remain). The egg substitute will smell slightly sweet and spicy. Refrigerate at least 15 minutes, or until cool, before using, or cover and refrigerate for up to two weeks.

Note: Flaxseed is available at health food stores and some supermarkets.

Makes about ⅔ cup

No added fat

Flax

A field of flax in full purple bloom? Irresistible! A bag of flaxseed in a health food store? Until now, a very tough sell. But that's about to change.

Shoppers in the new millennium may see flaxseed as an important new super food. Stocked inside this lowly seed are two impressive compounds looking more and more like foes of heart attacks, breast and colon cancer, arthritis, severe menstrual cramps, and even depression. What's mind-boggling is that flaxseed has more of these two compounds—lignans and alpha-linolenic acid—than any other food . . . by far.

In fact, flaxseed researcher Stephen Cunnane, Ph.D., associate professor of Nutritional Sciences at the University of Toronto, says, "There's nobody who won't benefit from adding flaxseed to his diet." If you're curious about how to do that, read on. Flaxseed is a winner that you'll want on your team.

Just the Flax, Ma'am

Each autumn, Canadian flax farmers, the world's top producers, harvest hard, shiny flaxseeds—usually brown but sometimes gold—shaped like diminutive sesame seeds. What's inside each seed could be better health, spelled F-L-A-X.

F is for fiber. It's amazing how much fiber a little flax contains. Just ¼ cup of ground flaxseed delivers 6 grams of fiber, as much fiber as 1½ cups of cooked oatmeal. Studies prove that when flaxseed is added to the diet, harmful low-density lipoprotein, or LDL, cholesterol drops, while good high-density lipoprotein, or HDL, cholesterol stays put, probably because of all that fiber (including the soluble kind). Regularity improves as well.

And most Americans need more fiber. We average less than 15 grams a day, about half the amount that health authorities recommend to help reduce the risk of colon cancer, heart disease, high blood pressure, and diabetes.

L is for lignans. Here's where the flaxseed story starts racking up major points. Lignans are tantalizing plant-based compounds that can shrink existing breast cancer and colon cancer tumors and stop new ones from getting started—at least in test-tube and animal studies. And flaxseed has staggering lignan levels. Many plant foods have some lignans, but flaxseed has at least 75 times more than any other. To get the lignans that are in just ¼ cup of flaxseed, you'd need to eat about 60 cups of fresh broccoli—or 100 slices of whole-wheat bread.

The discovery of flaxseed as a lignan storehouse came by sheer chance, says Kenneth Setchell, Ph.D., professor of pediatrics at Children's Hospital Medical Center in Cincinnati. In a study in 1978, he and his colleagues unexpectedly found lignan levels in one patient several hundred times higher than had ever been seen before. The patient, it turned out, baked his own bread—and always added flaxseed.

The first study testing lignans against cancer in humans is under way. One hundred women with breast cancer will eat a daily muffin with 25 grams of flaxseed to see if it might reduce the growth of their tumors between the time of diagnosis and surgery, according to study leader Lilian Thompson, Ph.D., professor of nutritional science at the University of Toronto. But remember one important point: Muffins are not a substitute for medical treatment. If you have breast cancer, seek or continue conventional care.

A is for alpha-linolenic acid. Mounting evidence suggests that you'll get considerable benefits from eating food that has more omega-3 fatty acids. This benign variety of fat, which is especially high in cold-water fish, has been found to reduce the incidence of heart attacks and to help ward off autoimmune diseases like rheumatoid arthritis, severe menstrual cramps, and maybe even depression. Many researchers tell us that modern diets—even healthy ones—are routinely deficient in omega-3's.

Once again, flaxseed turns out to be a mega-source, this time for the plant version of omega-3 called alpha-linolenic acid. The oil in flaxseed is about 50 percent alpha-linolenic acid. Canola and walnut oils, the next highest sources, have about 10 percent. But most foods have far less. It would take 25 cups of peanut butter, for example, to get the alpha-linolenic acid in just ¼ cup of ground flaxseed. Although the animal version of omega-3 fat, found in fish oil, packs the most punch, research confirms that alpha-linolenic acid confers omega-3 benefits, too. So, if you're a vegetarian or you don't eat fish regularly, says Dr. Cunnane, flaxseed is your best omega-3 bet.

To get the most omega-3's, look for flaxseed oil in health food stores. But to get the entire flax arsenal—omega-3's plus lignans and fiber—look for products that deliver the entire flaxseed. *Note:* You can use flaxseed, but not flaxseed oil, for baking. Under sustained heat, flaxseed oil (added as a separate ingredient) oxidizes and should not be consumed. But it is terrific in salad dressings or drizzled on pasta, steamed vegetables, or other foods after they are cooked.

X is for excellent. Should you consider adding flaxseed to your diet? "Absolutely," says Dr. Setchell. In terms of safety, flaxseed has been consumed since the Stone Age—a rather venerable track record. Ironically, most flaxseed is used today to make an inedible product—linseed oil, a component of paints and varnishes. (The word linseed by itself is simply an alternate word for flaxseed.) Linseed oil is oil that has been chemically

Fabulous Flaxseed Muffins

The expert cooks in *Prevention*'s test kitchen created this recipe to deliver 25 grams of flaxseed per muffin, the amount currently being tested against breast cancer.

        3   cups ground flaxseed
     1¼   cups flour
        1   tablespoon baking powder
      ¾   cup skim milk
      ½   cup egg substitute
   ⅓–½   cup light molasses
        2   tablespoons canola oil

Preheat the oven to 350°F.

In a large bowl, whisk together the flaxseed, flour, and baking powder. In a separate bowl, stir together the milk, egg substitute, molasses, and oil. Stir the milk mixture into the flaxseed mixture until just moistened.

Pour the batter into a 2¾" muffin pan coated with nonstick spray. Bake for about 18 minutes, or until the tops are lightly browned. The muffins can be frozen for use as needed.

Note: These muffins are higher in fat than what we usually recommend. However, nearly half the fat is alpha-linolenic acid—the plant version of omega-3, which is sorely missing in most diets.

Makes 12 muffins

Per muffin: 196 calories, 12.4 g. fat, 110 mg. sodium, 8.4 g. fiber, 25 g. flaxseed

extracted from flaxseeds and denatured—oxidized—which makes it unfit for human consumption.

Overcoming "Fear of Flax"

"Okay, but how does this stuff taste?" you must be thinking. The verdict: pleasantly nutty. To get health benefits, researchers estimate that you need anywhere from 6 grams to 25 grams a day (in ground flaxseed, that works out to 1 level measuring tablespoon up to ¼ cup). Because a few people are highly allergic to flax, start by using less than ¼ teaspoon a day, increasing gradually if no reactions occur.

Adding flax to your diet is easy. Here's how.

Try a sprinkle a day. At health food stores, look for pre-ground flaxseed (it's like cornmeal in consistency) with vitamins C and E added to stabilize it against oxidation. Sometimes small amounts of vitamin B_6 and zinc also are added, but flax researchers aren't convinced that these are necessary. Sprinkle one or more tablespoons in hot or cold cereal, yogurt, soup, or fruit juice. (Allow for extra calories and fat: Each tablespoon contains 25 calories, 2.5 grams of fat.) Once a package of pre-ground flaxseed is opened, keep it refrigerated; try to use within six months.

If you prefer to buy whole flaxseed, for maximum health benefits it should be ground in a coffee grinder or food processor—any whole seeds not crushed by your teeth in chewing will pass through you undigested. Use freshly ground flaxseed promptly.

Make your own treats. In blind taste tests among 90 college students, muffins and cookies with ground flaxseed in the recipe won out over plain muffins and cookies for flavor, tenderness, and color. So experiment using flaxseed in your own recipes.

Buy flax foods ready-made. In the United States, flaxseed is turning up at health food stores and in some Midwestern supermarkets, in breads and other products. In parts of Canada, flaxseed breads and breakfast cereals can also be found in supermarkets, bagel shops, and restaurants.

And finally, for some freshly baked flaxseed breads, muffins, and rolls delivered to your door by United Parcel Service, call Natural Ovens of Manitowoc, Wisconsin, at (800) 558-3535, Central time between 9:00 A.M. and 5:00 P.M.

One Week of Natural Healing

Andrew Weil, M.D., professor of herbalism and director of the Program of Integrative Medicine at the University of Arizona College of Medicine, near Tucson, is one of America's foremost experts on alternative medicine. In this excerpt from his book Eight Weeks to Optimum Health: A Proven Program for Taking Full Advantage of Your Body's Natural Healing Power, *Dr. Weil explains how to begin revamping your lifestyle.*

Congratulations! You are about to embark on an exciting and healthy adventure of restyling your life in order to attain optimum health.

I will give you specific directions for projects to do, as well as for changes to make in your diet and patterns of exercise. I will tell you about dietary supplements that are safe and effective, and I will also give you suggestions for taking advantage of the mind-body connection and for increasing spiritual energy.

First, I will outline the steps of this beginning week of the Eight-Week Program; then, I will present an extensive commentary on each step so that you will understand the reasons for doing them. Let's begin!

This Week's Projects: Sort, Toss, Get Going

• Start by going through your pantry and refrigerator to identify and discard common unhealthy foods. Throw out all oils other than olive oil and throw out any olive oil that smells old or rancid. Get rid of any margarine, solid vegetable shortenings, and products made with them (such as cookies and crackers). Also discard any products made with cottonseed oil. Read the labels of all food products so that you can dispose of any containing partially hydrogenated oils of any kind. If you do not have any extra-virgin olive oil on hand, buy a bottle and start using it. You might also want to buy a small bottle of organic, expeller-pressed canola oil from the health food store and some dark-roasted sesame oil from a Chinese or Japanese grocery store or the Asian-food section of the supermarket.

- Throw out any artificial sweeteners containing saccharin or aspartame and any products made with them.
- Throw out any products containing artificial coloring (indicated on the label by phrases like "color added," "artificially colored," or the name of a particular dye, such as "FD&C red #3").
- Make a commitment to read the labels of all the food products you buy. Pay special attention to the fat content, especially the saturated-fat content. I would like you to keep your total fat intake to about 20 to 25 percent of calories, and saturated-fat intake as low as possible. Do not buy products with labels that list more chemicals than recognizable ingredients.

Diet

- Start eating some fresh broccoli this week. If you like this vegetable and have favorite ways of preparing it, you know what to do. Otherwise, try the recipe on page 272.
- Eat salmon, sardines, or kippers at least once a week. (You will find some great, easy salmon recipes beginning on page 273.) If you do not want to eat fish, buy some flaxseeds at a health food store, grind them (directions are on page 271), and sprinkle them over your food once or twice a week.

Supplements

- Start taking vitamin C if you do not do so already: 1,000 to 2,000 milligrams with breakfast, another dose with dinner, and a third dose at bedtime, if convenient.

  Note: Some people have excessive flatulence or develop diarrhea when they take this much vitamin C in a day, so take less if you develop these symptoms.

Exercise

- Try to walk 10 minutes a day five days this week. If you are already on a program of aerobics exercise other than walking, do the walks in addition.

Mental/Spiritual

- Think about your own experiences of healing. Make a list of illnesses or injuries or problems that you have recovered from in the past two years. Note down anything you did to speed the healing process.
- Begin to practice the breath observation exercise on page 279 for 5 minutes every day.
- Buy some flowers to keep in your home, where you can enjoy them.

Dr. Weil Explains It All

I've asked you to clear out your pantry and refrigerator of unhealthy foods, beginning with fats and oils. Here is the rationale for doing so.

Stale fats are extremely unhealthy. On exposure to air, fats oxidize. Polyunsaturated fats oxidize more readily than monounsaturated ones, and monounsaturated fats oxidize faster than saturated ones.

Rates of oxidation increase with exposure to light and warmer temperatures. As oxidation progresses, fats become rancid, a condition easily detected by the human nose. Oxidized fats can damage DNA, promote the development of cancer, and speed up aging and degenerative changes in our tissues.

Always smell oils before you use them, discarding any if you can detect even a hint of rancidity. It is also a good idea to get in the habit of smelling foods that contain fat before you eat them, especially nuts, chips, and snack foods, to make sure that the oils have not oxidized. When you purchase oils, buy smaller rather than larger containers, keep them in the refrigerator, and use them up quickly.

The tendency to oxidize readily is the problem with most vegetable oils, particularly the polyunsaturated ones that fill the shelves of supermarkets: safflower, sunflower, corn, sesame, and soy. I recommend against using any of them.

The only exception I make is for the dark-roasted sesame oil that is a popular ingredient in Chinese and Japanese cuisines. Its flavor is so intense that it can be used to small amounts—from a few drops to a teaspoon or two at most—to season soups and stir-fries at the end of cooking; it can also be used to make a great low-fat salad dressing.

Dab on the Olive Oil

The best all-around oil to use is olive oil. Olive oil contains mostly monounsaturated fat, which seem much better for our bodies than either polyunsaturated or saturated fat.

We seem to be able to process oleic acid, the principal fatty acid in olive oil, better than any other fatty acid, and populations that rely on olive oil as their main dietary fat have lower rates of both heart disease and cancer than Americans and most Europeans do, even though their total fat intake is not that much lower.

Remember, olive oil is still fat; eating it immoderately can raise cholesterol and contribute to obesity. In moderation it is a healthy ingredient that can make food much more appealing. Buy a good brand of extra-virgin olive oil—the result of the first, gentle pressing of the olives—so that you can enjoy its rich flavor. Let your eye and nose guide you: The best olive oils are green or greenish yellow and have a delightful, fruity aroma.

Professional cooks often discourage you from cooking with the extra-virgin form because they say that it should be reserved for salads and special dishes. I disagree. As with all oils, keep this one in the refrigerator to protect it from light, heat, and resultant oxidation.

Olive oil will slowly solidify in the cold, but can easily be made pourable again by setting the bottle in hot water for a few minutes. (If you use it frequently, you can keep a small amount at room temperature for convenience.)

If you need to use oil in a dish you are preparing where the flavor of olive oil would be inappropriate, I suggest that you use canola oil, a neutral-flavored monounsaturated oil obtained from the seed of a plant related to mustard. In recent years, canola has acquired a reputation as a heart-healthy oil, but I consider it a distant runner-up to olive oil. Canola oil is not made up mostly of oleic acid, nor do we have epidemiological evidence, comparable to that for olive oil, of its association with good health in populations that use a lot of it.

In any case, the canola oil you will find in most grocery stores is not acceptable. It has been extracted with chemical solvents or by high-speed presses that generate high heat; both extraction methods alter fatty-acid chemistry in undesirable ways. (I will explain more about this when I tell you why you have to throw out any margarine you might have on hand.)

Furthermore, canola producers use a lot of pesticides on the crop, residues of which probably find their way into the final product. For these reasons, I recommend only organic, expeller-pressed canola oil, which you are most likely to find in health food stores.

Leave Margarine Behind

On to margarine. It has two strikes against it that render it unfit for consumption by anyone wanting to attain optimum health.

First, the process of hardening vegetable oils to create solid spreads increases the percentage of saturated fat and thereby diminishes any advantage over butter in the realm of cardiovascular friendliness.

Second, and of even greater concern to me because it is a danger less recognized by doctors, the process of artificially hydrogenating oils deforms fatty acids, creating an unnatural species called *trans*-fatty acids, or TFAs. Putting TFAs into your body may unbalance the hormonal systems that regulate healing, lead to the construction of defective cell membranes, and encourage the development of cancer.

If it comes to a choice between butter and margarine, always take butter. But I hope that you will be able to reduce your butter consumption as well because it is one of the highest sources of saturated fat in our diets, clearly implicated in atherosclerosis and arterial disease. It is possible to learn to enjoy really good bread with nothing on it, and to enjoy vegetables without butter or margarine.

If you must put fat on bread, try a little olive oil or some mashed, seasoned avocado (a source of monounsaturated oil). You can also find in the refrigerators of health food stores new emulsified vegetable-oil spreads made without heat or hydrogenation.

The Solid Case against Hardened Fats

For the same reasons that I reject margarine as a food, I also urge you to avoid all other sources of artificially hardened fats.

Solid vegetable shortening is easy to do without. Much harder are all of the commercial products made with partially hydrogenated oils. Manufacturers like these unnatural fats because they oxidize less quickly than liquid oil, yielding longer shelf life.

No matter how good the oils are that go into the process of partial hydrogenation, what comes out is unnatural and unhealthy, since it is full of TFAs. I predict that accumulating medical evidence about the harmfulness of partially hydrogenated oils will eventually force them out of food products.

In the meantime, I cannot urge you too strongly to read labels carefully and reject all products containing them. Partially hydrogenated oils are ubiquitous in snack foods, baked goods, cookies, crackers, spreads, and many other items in grocery stores and supermarkets.

I've asked you to avoid cottonseed oil and anything made with it because it has too high a percentage of saturated fat, may contain natural toxins, and probably has unacceptably high levels of pesticide residues, since cotton is not classified as a food crop and farmers use many agrichemicals when growing it. Again, get in the habit of reading labels carefully when you shop for food.

Fats are one of the three "macronutrients" we eat, the others being proteins and carbohydrates. There is now a great deal of information about how the amount and kind of fat we eat affects our health, and I will summarize some of that information in the commentary that follows the one-week instruction. I will also give you the most up-to-date facts I have about choosing proteins and carbohydrates wisely in order to protect and enhance your capacity for natural healing.

Reject All Artificial Ingredients

The other products that I asked you to throw away this first week are foods containing artificial sweeteners, artificial colors, and large numbers of chemical additives. These substances do not require lengthy comment.

There is not a shred of evidence that the availability of artificial, noncaloric sweeteners has helped anyone lose weight—the main reason for their popularity—and enough evidence of potential harm to exclude them from a healthy diet. Saccharin, cyclamates, and aspartame (NutraSweet) all taste funny and disturb physiology in some people (causing headaches and menstrual dysfunction, for example). Some experts suspect them of promoting cancer and having toxic effects on the nervous system. You are much better off eating moderate amounts of sugar than any of these unnatural compounds.

Similarly, the chemicals used to dye foods, drugs, and cosmetics are a suspect group of highly reactive molecules that may interact with DNA in ways that increase mutation and malignant transformation cells. Read labels and avoid them. I do not object to natural coloring agents like annatto (yellow/orange), beet (red/purple), carotene (yellow/orange), chlorella (green), and caramel (brown).

Become a Broccoli Believer

The dietary changes recommended in the Eight-Week Program are intended to move you in the direction of eating less fat (especially less saturated fat), less animal protein, more whole grains and other complex carbohydrates, and more fresh fruits and vegetables.

This week I have asked you to eat some fresh broccoli, one of the most healthful members of the cabbage family, or crucifers. (The name means "crossbearer," referring to the pattern formed by the flower petals of plants in this group.) Cruciferous vegetables have significant anti-cancer properties; broccoli is most effective in this regard, and one of its most important constituents, sulphoraphane, is even sold in tablet form ("broccoli in a pill") in health food stores.

Of course, isolated sulphoraphane is no more broccoli in a pill than beta-carotene is a carrot. Broccoli has many nutrients and protective compounds in it as well as fiber. It also tastes good and is a source of pleasure in the diet if it is well-prepared.

I have in my life encountered plenty of poorly prepared broccoli, which is anything but a source of pleasure. The easiest way to ruin this vegetable is to overcook it, turning it into a yellowish green, malodorous mush. I am sure that most people who think they do not like broccoli know it only in that form.

I do not recommend eating broccoli raw because it does not taste especially good that way and may be less digestible. Perfectly cooked broccoli should be beautifully bright green and crisp-tender; my family and I like it really crunchy. That might require only 5 minutes of cooking or less, meaning you cannot put the pot on the stove and ignore it.

Broccoli stalks are delicious if they are peeled properly, and a simple technique—peeling to beneath the fibrous layer—also renders the smaller stems more tender. It is true that the preparation of fresh vegetables takes time—not very much, in the case of broccoli—but what it really takes is knowledge of how to maximize flavor, appearance, and nutritive value.

I hope that you will begin to experiment with new vegetables and ways of preparing them. Scientific evidence for the protective effects of vegetables on health is very strong.

Learn to Appreciate Fish

The other dietary change that I have asked you to make this week is to begin eating some fish if you do not already do so. The kinds of fish I have recommended are oily fish from cold, Northern waters: salmon, sardines, kippers, mackerel. Salmon is easily available fresh; the others you will find in cans.

My reason for including these fish in the Eight-Week Program is that they are excellent sources of omega-3 fatty acids, special fats that have beneficial effects on many body functions. For example, they inhibit the clotting tendency of the blood, reducing the risk of heart attack. They improve the serum-lipid profile (blood fats), and they modify the production of hormones called eicosanoids that control tissue growth and repair, reducing excessive inflammation and promoting healing.

If you do not want to eat fish, there are some vegetarian sources of omega-3's that I will tell you about in a moment, but be aware that including some fish in your diet may improve your health in other ways. In general, fish-eating populations have higher longevity and lower rates of disease than non-fish-eating populations, and the differences may not have to do only with intake of omega-3 fatty acids.

I happen to like salmon a lot and will give you my favorite ways of preparing it beginning on page 273. Be aware that wild salmon is more nutritious, having a significantly higher content of omega-3's than farmed salmon. You can find canned kippers (smoked herring fillets) with or without added salt in all supermarkets. There are many preparations of sardines available as well. Avoid those packed in any oils other than sardine oil or olive oil; my preference is for water-packed ones.

If you do get an oil-packed variety, drain off as much oil as you can before using the fish in order to get rid of as many extra fat calories as you can. Fresh mackerel is delicious but available only seasonally; most stores stock canned mackerel fillets, sometimes in tomato—or another flavorful—sauce.

Consider the Flax

Here are your options for getting omega-3's in your diet without eating fish. You can buy capsules of fish oils in drugstores and health food stores, but I advise you not to use them. It is not clear that they reproduce the benefits of whole fish, and they may contain toxic contaminants.

Instead, I suggest adding homemade flax meal to your diet, since this is a cheap and convenient source of the fatty acids you want. Buy whole flaxseeds at a health food store. Keep them in the refrigerator and grind ½ cup or so at a time, using a blender or coffee grinder.

Ground flax has a nutty taste that is quite good added to cereals, salads, potatoes, rice, or cooked vegetables. A tablespoon of the meal once a day will give you a good ration of omega-3's. Be aware that flaxseeds are high in fiber and will increase the bulk of stools; in some individuals they may exert a laxative effect. Most people find this effect welcome, but some do not. If it bothers you, eat less.

You will see dark plastic bottles of flaxseed oil in the refrigerator and freezer cases of health food stores. I think that flax meal is preferable, being cheaper and tastier. Flax oil oxidizes very readily and, unless it is handled and packaged with great care, develops the unpleasant taste of oil paint, a sign of rancidity and hardly a welcome addition to food.

Other specialty oils that provide omega-3's but are not yet generally available come from the seeds of hemp and hops. Canola and soy oils are the only common vegetable oils that have omega-3's, though not nearly as much as flax.

There is also one vegetable that contains omega-3's: purslane (*Portulaca oleracea*), sometimes eaten as a wild green in the United States but more commonly despised by gardeners as an invasive weed. In other parts of the world, people cultivate purslane and like it as a vegetable. Greeks often add it to soups, for example, and some experts think that it contributes to the heart-healthiness of Mediterranean diets. Specialty seed catalogs offer improved varieties of purslane for home gardens. If you like to produce some of your own food, consider this easy-to-grow creeping plant with small, succulent leaves.

On the following pages are some recipes to help you implement the dietary recommendations of this first week of the program. (All recipes in this chapter are meant to yield three to four servings).

Dr. Andrew Weil's Favorite Low-Fat Salad Dressing

Seasoned rice-wine vinegar (see note)
1 **teaspoon dark-roasted sesame oil**

Pour enough vinegar over prepared salad greens in a serving bowl to coat them lightly. Add the oil. (Remember, its flavor is so intense that a little goes a remarkably long way.)

Toss well and serve.

Note: Seasoned rice-wine vinegar can be bought in a Japanese grocery store or the Asian-food section of a supermarket; it is seasoned with sugar and salt. Avoid brands that contain MSG (monosodium glutamate). You can also buy plain rice-wine vinegar and season it yourself with sugar or honey and salt to taste.

This couldn't be easier. For variety, you can try adding a clove of garlic, crushed, to the vinegar before you pour it over the greens.

Broccoli

Here is my preferred preparation of this wonderfully healthful vegetable.

1 **large bunch broccoli**
1 **tablespoon extra-virgin olive oil**
  Salt
  Several cloves garlic, chopped
  Red-pepper flakes (optional)

Trim the bottoms of the broccoli stalks and discard. Cut off the main stem of each stalk, peel it to beneath the fibrous layer, and cut the flesh into edible chunks. Separate the head of broccoli into bite-size pieces and peel a bit of the skin from the small stems to make them more tender.

Wash the broccoli in cold water, drain, and place in a pot with ¼ cup cold water, the oil, salt, to taste, and the garlic. Add a pinch or more of the red-pepper flakes if you want a spicy dish.

Bring to a boil, cover tightly, and let steam until the broccoli is bright green and very crunchy-tender, no more than 5 minutes. Remove with a slotted spoon and serve at once.

Note: You can also add the broccoli (with any remaining liquid) to cooked pasta (I prefer penne or rigatoni), seasoning with grated Parmesan cheese if you like.

Grilled or Broiled Salmon

1   **cup sake**
½   **cup natural soy sauce, or tamari**
1   **tablespoon grated fresh ginger**
2   **cloves fresh garlic, mashed**
1   **tablespoon dark brown sugar**
    Salmon fillets (allow 6 ounces per person)
    Lemon wedges (optional)

Prepare a marinade by mixing the sake (Japanese rice wine), soy sauce (a reduced-sodium variety if you prefer), ginger, garlic, and brown sugar.

Rinse the fish fillets under cold water. Place them in a glass or ceramic dish and pour on the marinade. Cover and let marinate in the refrigerator for 1 to 3 hours, spooning the liquid over any exposed parts of the fish once or twice.

Prepare the grill or preheat the broiler to high heat.

Drain the fish and place on foil on the grill or oven rack. Cook until desired doneness, but do not overcook. Serve at once, with lemon wedges (if using). Makes a great meal with rice and a cooked vegetable or salad.

Easy Poached Salmon

    Salmon fillets (allow 6 ounces per person)
1 **carrot, sliced**
1 **small onion, sliced**
1 **stalk celery, sliced**
2 **slices lemon**
    Several sprigs of parsley
6 **Turkish bay leaves (see note)**
    Salt
1 **cup dry white wine**
    Juice of ½ lemon

Cut the fish fillets into individual portions.

Place in a medium saucepan the carrots, onions, celery, lemon slices, parsley, and bay leaves.

Add the fish, cold water to cover, salt, to taste, wine, and lemon juice. Bring the pot to a boil, uncovered.

Adjust the heat to simmer and let the fish cook for 5 minutes.

Turn off the heat and leave the fish undisturbed for 10 minutes. Then remove it carefully to a serving platter; the salmon will be perfectly done. It is delicious served either hot or cold.

Note: Turkish bay leaves are preferred. If using California bay leaves instead, use half of a large leaf.

Salmon in Parchment

This is an easy and elegant main-dish preparation. It requires cooking parchment, which you will find in rolls or sheets at kitchen-supply stores.

    Thin spaghetti
    Olive oil
    Salt
    Fresh dill or parsley, chopped

Fresh vegetables

Salmon fillet

Dijon mustard

Preheat the oven to 400°F.

Cook the spaghetti until just done (al dente), drain, toss with a bit of oil, salt, and dill (or parsley).

Prepare a garnish of the fresh vegetables: carrot and zucchini matchsticks, asparagus tips, snow or snap pea pods, or the like.

Rinse the fish fillet, cut in individual portions, and pat dry. Spread the top of each one with the mustard.

For each person, place a serving of the pasta on a sheet of baking parchment, top with a fillet, add the vegetables, and twist the corners of the parchment together to seal into a pouch.

Place the pouches in the middle of the oven and bake for 10 minutes. Serve immediately in the sealed pouches, opening them just before eating.

C Is the First Letter in the Supplement Alphabet

You are to start taking vitamin C this week, the first of four antioxidant supplements making up a formula that I take myself and recommend for everyone. Maybe you already take vitamin C and other dietary supplements. If you do not, here are the reasons to begin doing so.

Almost all animals make vitamin C in their bodies. Only human beings, other primates, and a very few other species have lost this ability and need to get the vitamin every day from dietary sources, principally fresh fruits and vegetables.

You need certain levels of vitamin C to build strong connective tissue, including the linings of coronary arteries, and to allow the healing system to repair wounds. I believe that higher doses can encourage healing on all levels as well as help the body protect itself from oxidative damage by free radicals, the highly reactive molecules generated by exposure to chemical and energetic toxins as well as by normal metabolism.

As an example of vitamin C's effect on the healing system, let me tell a story that happened just a few weeks ago. The older brother of a friend of mine underwent surgery for removal of portions of his stomach and esophagus. Before he entered the hospital, he asked me what he could do to speed his recovery, and I gave him two standard recommendations.

First, I told him to get permission from the anesthesiologist to wear a headset during the operation and have an audiotape made of suggestions for success of the surgery and a rapid recovery with minimal pain. This would serve two purposes: It would block out any conversation in the operating room that would put unwanted ideas in his mind, and it would take advantage of the mind's influence on the healing system in a state when the unconscious mind readily accepts suggestion.

My second recommendation was to tell his surgeon that he wanted high doses of vitamin C put into his intravenous (IV) drip from the time he went into surgery until the IV was removed: 20 grams in every 24-hour period. I also told him not to expect compliance with this request; in my experience most hospitals will not honor it.

This patient took a very aggressive stance with his doctors and insisted on the intravenous vitamin C. He got it. When the surgeon examined him several days after the operation, he told the patient that he had never seen such rapid healing from a surgical wound and was so impressed that he would begin ordering IV vitamin C in all of his cases.

Supplemental vitamin C is nontoxic. It does not promote the formation of kidney stones, as some have charged, but it can disturb bowel function in very high dosage.

If you take increasing doses of this vitamin, you will at some point reach your level of bowel tolerance, marked initially by flatulence and then by diarrhea. You will want to stay below the dose that causes these effects, and since the level varies greatly from person to person, you may have to experiment. I recommend 1 to 2 grams (1,000 to 2,000 milligrams) two or three times a day, for a total daily dose of 2 to 6 grams (2,000 to 6,000 milligrams). If you can remember to take this vitamin three times a day (say, at breakfast, dinner, and bedtime), that will keep it available to your body all the time. At least try to take it twice a day, at 12-hour intervals.

I like to use an effervescent, powdered form of vitamin C that is nonacidic. (This product, called C–Salts, is available from Wholesale Nutrition, P.O. Box 3345, Saratoga, CA 95070-9942.) Do not use sweet, chewable tablets (bad for the teeth) or huge, hard tablets (may not dissolve), or fancy brands that are very expensive.

Do not expect immediate effects from vitamin C, although it may

decrease frequency of colds and reduce easy bruising in some people. You are taking it as a part of a long-range strategy to protect your healing system and enhance its functioning so it will be able to maintain your day-to-day well-being and be ready to serve you in case of illness.

Walk This Way

Exercise is a key component of a healthy lifestyle. You cannot enjoy optimal health and healing if you are sedentary. You may have heard that walking is the best exercise. It's true, and I'm asking you to do a lot of it in this Eight-Week Program. Here are the advantages of walking.

- You already know how to do it.
- You can do it anywhere.
- It requires no equipment, just a good pair of shoes.
- It caries the least risk of injury of any form of exercise.
- It can provide a complete workout, equal to or better than any other activity.
- It will satisfy all your exercise requirements throughout your life, even into old age.

Many fitness buffs look down on walking as being tame compared with running, playing competitive sports, or driving oneself to sweaty exhaustion on stationary bicycles and other aerobic torture devices. It's not so. I have seen people attain maximum fitness through walking alone; they did it conscientiously and regularly and did enough of it to take full advantage of its wonderful conditioning effect on the body, and they used no other form of physical activity to get to their goal. I have also seen very obese people reach their optimal weights in several months by walking every day in combination with sensible dietary modification.

My preference is to walk outside in beautiful surroundings, but if I'm in a city, I will gladly walk around it as much as possible, and if I encounter bad weather, I might just walk back and forth in a shopping mall or try to find a gym where I can walk on a treadmill. For maximum cardiovascular benefit, you should try to include some up-hill walking—long, moderate, sustained grades are terrific—or walk fast enough to get your heart rate up. You can buy a miniature heart-rate monitor to wear like a wristwatch (along with a band that straps around your chest), or you can learn to take your pulse at the wrist for 15 seconds and multiply by 4 to get beats per minute. The Target Heart Rate Zone (THRZ), in which

maximal aerobic conditioning takes place and fat burning occurs, can be calculated by a not-too-complicated formula. First, determine your Predicted Maximal Heart Rate (PMHR). For physically inactive men, and women of any activity level, the PMHR is 220 minus your age; for physically active men it is 205 minus your age. THRZ is then 65 to 75 percent of your PMHR. For example, I am now 54 and physically active, so my PMHR is 151. My THRZ is 98 to 113, and a 15-second pulse rate in this zone would be one-quarter of those figures, or 24 to 28. In general, if you are exercising about your THRZ, you will be too aerobically stressed to carry on a conversation, and if you are exercising below it, you will not notice your heart and breath going significantly faster than normal.

Sometimes I like to walk alone and be with my thoughts and nature. Sometimes I like to walk with a friend and pass the time in conversation. Sometimes I carry a portable cassette player and listen to spirited music with a beat that keeps my feet moving quickly. Cassette players and tapes have transformed walking for many; I know people who like to listen to books on tape or foreign-language lessons while they do their daily walks.

I've asked you to begin this practice with a 10-minute daily walk (if you are already walking this much or more, keep at it), and I want you to do it even if you have some other exercise routine because I feel that walking offers benefits that other forms of activity do not, such as conditioning rhythms in the brain in response to the coordinated motions of the arms and legs.

If you are not used to walking, be sure to wear the right shoes. I recommend running shoes with good cushioning in the insoles; many brands are available at athletic-supply stores. You will also find special double-layer socks that prevent blisters and wick away perspiration from your feet. Think about where you are going to walk and when and how you are going to build this activity into your daily routine. I like to take morning walks, before breakfast, but if I miss the chance, I'm just as happy to walk at the end of the day.

Nurture Your Mind and Spirit

The recommendations that fall under this heading are most important. If you have read my earlier writings on health, you know that I am a strong proponent of mind-body medicine, who believes that illness in the physical body is often the result of imbalance in the mind or the spiritual

realm. For your healing system to function optimally, you must address those areas of your being as well as look after the needs of your body. I will ease you into this area of work with practices that are gentle and interesting, that I think you will enjoy, and that, despite their simplicity, are profoundly effective.

This week, I have asked you to think about your own experiences of healing—from any recent illnesses, injuries, or problems (emotional as well as physical). I want you to focus attention on healing because the way to experience more of something you want is to become more conscious of it. If you like to keep journals or diaries, you might want to get a notebook in which to record these experiences and new ones. It is a way to build up confidence in the power of spontaneous healing inside you.

Next, I have asked you to begin working with your breath, a practice that will develop as you progress through the Eight-Week Program. I have written extensively about the healing power of breath in other books. Suffice it to say that breath is the link between the body and mind and between the conscious and unconscious mind. It is the master key to the control of emotions and to the operations of the involuntary nervous system.

Moreover, breath represents the movement of spirit in matter. Turning your attention to your breath moves you naturally toward relaxation and meditation and puts you in conscious touch with your vital, nonphysical essence.

The simplest technique of breath work is simply to observe it, to do nothing other than follow the breath cycle with your observing mind, without trying to influence it in any way. Here are a couple formal instructions.

1. Sit in a comfortable position with your back straight and your eyes lightly closed, having loosened any tight clothing.
2. Focus your attention on your breathing, and follow the contours of the cycle through inhalation and exhalation, noting, if you can, the points at which one phase changes into the other.

Do this for 5 minutes once a day. Your goal is simply to keep your attention on the breath cycle and observe. No matter how the breath changes, even if the excursions become very small, just continue to follow them. This is a basic form of meditation, a relaxation method, and a way to begin to harmonize body, mind, and spirit.

Finally, this week, I have asked you to buy some fresh flowers to keep in your home, where you can enjoy them. I do not think much commentary is required. Flowers manifest the beauty and wonder of nature and delight the senses. It feels good to be around them. They raise our spirits.

That is all the information you need to go through the first week of the Eight-Week Program.

Supplements Made Simple

So how do you find the best supplements if you don't happen to have a Ph.D. in nutrition and a full weekend to spare doing research? Help is here.

Walk into any health food store or even your neighborhood pharmacy, and you can quickly be entangled in a confusing jungle of vitamins and minerals. Don't give up. Picking a supplement is actually easy—really, it is.

To help you make your choice, here's a selection of the nine key nutrients that you need to zero in on. Why these nine? These are the ones that get shortchanged in the typical American diet, according to top nutritional experts. The more of the following nine nutrients that a multivitamin/mineral supplement contains in levels close to experts' recommendations, the more complete it is.

Note: If you're pregnant, be sure to check with your doctor before adding any of these key nutrients to your diet.

Iron

This should be the first item that you check in a multi, since how much you need differs depending on your age and gender. Find a multi with the iron level that you want before you spend time checking other nutrients.

What to look for: Premenopausal women should look for up to 18 milligrams, which is 100 percent of the Daily Value (DV). Adult men and menopausal women should look for up to 9 milligrams (50 percent of the DV).

What the label won't tell you: Premenopausal women having periods lose iron each month and may need the help of a supplement to replace it. But women not having periods and adult men lose little iron normally. Since some research indicates that excess iron raises risks of heart disease and colon cancer, many experts now advise men and menopausal women to look for supplements with no iron or low iron. (Check your breakfast cereal; some are heavily fortified with iron. Take that into account when you select a multi.)

Be aware: Unless you're diagnosed with iron-deficiency anemia, there's no reason to take levels above 100 percent of the DV.

Vitamin A/Beta-Carotene

What to look for: Find a multi with 5,000 international units (IU), which is 100 percent of the DV.

What the label won't tell you: In most multis, the vitamin A is a mix of preformed vitamin A and its precursor, beta-carotene. Not all multis tell you how much comes from each. But even if a multi is all preformed vitamin A or all beta-carotene, 5,000 IU is considered a very safe level of each.

Be aware: Don't supplement above 10,000 IU—and most doctors advise that pregnant women should not go above 5,000 IU because too much preformed vitamin A can be toxic or cause birth defects. Can you get too much beta-carotene? Studies show that people with diets high in beta-carotene have lower risks of heart disease and cancer. But in two studies of long-term smokers, those taking high-dose beta-carotene supplements (25 milligrams or more) developed more lung cancer. Until more is known, a reasonable limit for beta-carotene from supplements (not food) is 6 milligrams. (That's what you'd get if 10,000 IU of vitamin A were all from beta-carotene.)

Vitamin D

What to look for: Try to get 400 IU (100 percent of the DV).

What the label won't tell you: Our bodies can manufacture vitamin D from the action of sunlight on the skin, but experts believe that many people (especially the elderly and those who routinely use sunblock) may not be exposed to enough sun.

Be aware: Don't get more than 600 IU of vitamin D a day from supplements plus fortified foods. Be sure to count vitamin D from milk (100 IU per 8-ounce glass or per ⅓ cup nonfat milk powder) or fortified breakfast cereal (amounts vary).

Vitamin B₆

What to look for: Try to get 2 milligrams (100 percent of the DV).

What the label won't tell you: American women's diets appear to be routinely low in B_6 (and for some women, oral contraceptives may increase the need). Low intakes are linked to higher levels of heart attack risk and poorer immune functioning in older people.

Be aware: Don't overdo B_6 (or any other vitamin or mineral, for that matter). Megadoses of 100 milligrams are associated with nerve damage. Problems also have been reported at intakes of 50 milligrams. Reports of high doses of vitamin B_6 relieving carpal tunnel syndrome or premenstrual syndrome have not been confirmed by research.

Folic Acid (or Folate)

What to look for: Try to get 400 micrograms, which is 100 percent of the DV. This may be listed as 0.4 milligram, which is the same as 400 micrograms.

What the label won't tell you: Studies prove that women taking supplements with 400 micrograms of folic acid prior to and in the first weeks of pregnancy give birth to fewer babies with serious brain and spine defects. There's strong indication that higher intakes of folic acid may help reduce risks of heart disease (by reducing blood levels of a substance called homocysteine) and colon cancer. But it's difficult to get 400 micrograms in your diet unless you choose several rich vegetable sources every day— such as lentils, spinach, kidney beans, asparagus, and chickpeas. (Folic acid is also found in animal sources such as chicken and beef liver, but unfortunately, these are too high in fat to include in most diets.)

Be aware: The U.S. Public Health Service has urged doctors to tell their patients about the proven and potential benefits of supplements containing 400 micrograms of folic acid—a nutrient that helps boost immunity.

Magnesium

What to look for: Try to get 100 milligrams (25 percent of the DV). That's the most you'll find in any single-dose multi supplement (more would make a pill that's too big to swallow). In a divided-dose multi, look for up to 400 milligrams (100 percent of the DV) in the day's total.

What the label won't tell you: Americans routinely eat far less than 100 percent of the DV of this intriguing mineral, which has been linked to protection from diabetes, osteoporosis, atherosclerosis, hypertension (high blood pressure), and migraine headaches.

Be aware: Excess magnesium can lead to diarrhea. Those with abnormal kidney function should not supplement magnesium without a doctor's supervision.

Zinc

What to look for: Try to get 15 milligrams (100 percent of the DV).

What the label won't tell you: Surveys show that this may be the mineral most lacking in Americans' diets. Zinc is necessary for a strong immune system and proper wound healing.

Be aware: Don't take supplements with more than 15 milligrams a day. Too much zinc—in one study, 50 milligrams to 75 milligrams a day—can backfire and lower "good" high-density lipoprotein, or HDL, cholesterol.

Copper

What to look for: Try to get 2 milligrams (100 percent of the DV).

What the label won't tell you: Here's another mineral that the average diet runs low on. Copper plays a role in bone and heart health, blood sugar regulation, and iron use.

Be aware: If your supplement has zinc, make sure that it has copper, too. Elevating zinc intake without taking in enough copper can suppress copper absorption.

Chromium

What to look for: Try to get 50 micrograms to 200 micrograms, a safe and adequate range set by the National Research Council.

What the label won't tell you: Research indicates that it may be difficult to get even the minimum amount of chromium that we need from food. This important mineral helps the body handle blood sugar; low levels of chromium may increase the risk of adult-onset (Type II) diabetes.

Note: You may not see a percent of DV for chromium; instead, there may be an asterisk (*) on some food labels that indicates "Daily Value not established." Though the Food and Drug Administration has set a DV for chromium of 120 micrograms, it may not be shown yet on some brands of supplements.

Be aware: Most studies do not support claims that extra chromium helps with weight loss or building muscle.

Consider Some Single Supplements, Too

If other vitamins and minerals are present in a multi, consider them nice to have but not necessary. For most of these it's preferable if levels stay in the range of 100 percent of the DV or lower. (People over the age of 60, however, may want to take extra vitamin B_{12}—from 200 percent to 500 percent of the DV—to make up for problems they might have absorbing vitamin B_{12} from food. But check with your doctor first.)

While the nine nutrients mentioned earlier are what you should look for in a multi—according to experts—there are three more that should be taken as single supplements. Most people need vitamin C, vitamin E, and calcium in amounts that you won't find in the standard single-dose multi supplement. Here's a closer look at this vital trio.

Vitamin C

The dose: Consider taking 200 to 500 milligrams of this antioxidant vitamin as a single supplement. Otherwise, make sure that your multi has at least 60 milligrams (100 percent of the DV).

The evidence: A study at the National Institutes of Health (NIH) in Bethesda, Maryland, found that we need 200 milligrams of vitamin C to keep blood cells at 85 percent saturation level. For 95 percent saturation, we need 400 to 500 milligrams. Researchers conclude that the current DV of 60 milligrams may be too low.

People with diets high in vitamin C have lower rates of cancer and heart disease. Although this is not yet proven, some studies hint that vitamin C supplements may help lower risk of cataracts as well as help those with diabetes.

What to look for: Find a vitamin C supplement in 100-, 250-, or 500-millgram tablets. Or find chewable tablets (to protect tooth enamel, chew only one a day), effervescent tablets, or powder that dissolves in water. You may find 100 milligrams or more of vitamin C in some multis.

Natural versus synthetic: Your body doesn't know the difference between vitamin C derived from rose hips or a laboratory.

Best way to take: Divide your dose in two; take half in the morning and half at night. After 12 hours, your body returns to presaturation levels, no matter what amount of vitamin C you've taken.

Can you get 200 to 500 milligrams of vitamin C from food? It's possible, if you eat lots of fruits and vegetables rich in vitamin C. An 8-ounce glass of orange juice from concentrate, for example, has 100 milligrams. A cup of fresh strawberries has 85 milligrams. One-half cup of frozen broccoli, cooked, has 40 milligrams.

Be aware: Although 1,000 milligrams of vitamin C yielded 100 percent saturation of blood cells in the NIH study, some research suggests that taking that much vitamin C may increase risk of kidney stones. Doctors warn that amounts over 1,200 milligrams per day can be toxic, and diarrhea may occur at intakes of several thousand milligrams.

Vitamin E

The dose: Consider taking 100 to 400 IU of this antioxidant vitamin. Most multis supply only about 30 IU (100 percent of the DV), much less than the levels that some research indicates may fight illness, especially heart disease. If you don't take extra vitamin E, make sure that your multi has at least 30 IU.

The evidence: Among the best indication that extra E may help is a British study of more than 2,000 men and women with narrowed coronary arteries. Participants took either 400 IU of E, 800 IU, or a placebo. After 18 months, vitamin E–takers (of either dose) lowered their chances of getting a nonfatal heart attack by 75 percent. Other research suggests that extra vitamin E may reduce risk of cataracts and some cancers and may help people who have diabetes.

What to look for: Find a vitamin E supplement in 100-, 200-, or 400-IU capsules. They're also available in chewable or liquid form.

Natural versus synthetic: Though natural vitamin E is more bioactive in the body than synthetic vitamin E, the difference in potency is taken into account in the international unit. That means that 100 IU of synthetic vitamin E is as potent as 100 IU of natural vitamin E. Most research, by the way, uses synthetic. To know which type your supplement has, read the list of ingredients. Natural vitamin E may be listed as "d-alpha-tocopherol" on the label, while synthetic is listed as "d,l-alpha-tocopherol."

Best way to take: Vitamin E is best taken with a meal that contains at least a little fat, to help with absorption.

Can you get 100 to 400 IU of vitamin E from food? Hardly! You would need 2 cups of corn oil, one of the best sources, to get 100 IU.

Be aware: If you're on blood-thinning medication or at risk for uncontrolled bleeding, talk with your doctor before taking a vitamin E supplement.

Calcium

The dose: Depending on the calcium in your diet, consider single supplements containing 500 to 1,000 milligrams of this crucial bone protector.

The evidence: It surprises many people that single-dose multi supplements are never complete with 100 percent of the DV for calcium (1,000 milligrams). In fact, that would be impossible—all that calcium would make a single tablet too big to swallow. Some single-dose multis do have about 200 milligrams. But since surveys show that many diets lag well behind recommended levels, a separate calcium supplement is worth considering.

What to look for: Calcium supplements are available in capsules and chewable tablets. Supplements made from calcium carbonate deliver the most calcium per tablet, so you'll have fewer pills to swallow (or tablets to chew). It also makes calcium carbonate supplements the least expensive, as a rule. Unfortunately, not all supplement labels make it easy to determine the source of the calcium. Some products use bonemeal, oyster shell, or dolomite, a natural mineral containing both calcium and magnesium. Sometimes oyster-shell calcium is identified only as "natural" calcium carbonate, and the words "oyster shell" do not appear on the label. Because there is no standard format, you may have to shop around to find calcium carbonate supplements.

Natural versus synthetic: In a 1993 study, it was found that natural supplements made from oyster shells, dolomite, and especially bonemeal contain levels of lead that greatly exceeded the lead in the quantity of milk supplying an equal amount of calcium. Most experts consider these levels unwise for children. For adults, who want to keep lead intake as low as possible, a nonnatural calcium supplement is the best choice. If a calcium carbonate product doesn't say "natural" or "oyster shell" on the label, it has been made from limestone refined in a laboratory. These nonnatural products contain some lead but not nearly as much as some natural calicum supplements.

Best way to take: With meals, all calcium supplements seem to be absorbed about the same. In addition, the potential benefits of calcium in reducing heart disease, blood pressure, and colon cancer may involve its interacting with other nutrients in food. But if it is more convenient for you to take supplements between meals, such as at bedtime, do it. Of the calcium supplements, calcium citrate is the best at being absorbed without food, especially by people over 60.

Can you get 500 to 1,000 milligrams of calcium from food? Frankly, unless you are a milk-lover, reaching the recommended levels of calcium intake through diet alone takes careful planning. It can be done but too often isn't.

Be aware: Diets high in calcium may increase your risk of developing kidney stones. If you're being treated for kidney stones, check with your doctor before taking calcium supplements.

The Wellness within Us

Science has discovered a link between religious commitment and better health, according to Herbert Benson, M.D., president of the Mind/Body Institute and director of behavioral medicine at Beth Israel Deaconess Medical Center/Harvard Medical School. In this excerpt from his book Timeless Healing, *Dr. Benson provides his perspective on the ways healing sometimes occurs in our lives.*

At one time or another, I'm sure that nearly everyone experiences extraordinary and magical events, the converging of time and circumstance so logic-defiant that one cannot help but feel these events were divinely directed.

It could be a chance reunion with a long-lost friend, a life change that comes at precisely the time you need it, or an image you see in a cloud formation. It could be a clergy person's sermon that seems eerily relevant to the problems you've been facing, something as dramatic as hearing a voice speak to you inspirationally, or as quiet as a bliss that envelops you suddenly.

Whatever the form, the more the incident means to us, the more we attach sacred status to it in our lives. We shake our heads, asking, "What are the chances?" all the while feeling a profound reverberation within that perhaps life is not random, that perhaps these are tangible signs that a mystical force contours our lives.

But it's possible that the reverberation you feel within when an experience you deem magical or spiritual occurs may not be just emotional but physical as well. Not only did my research—and that of my colleagues—reveal that 25 percent of people feel more spiritual as the result of the elicitation of the relaxation response, but it showed that those same people have fewer medical symptoms than do those who reported no increase in spirituality from the elicitation.

Faith Bolsters the Relaxation Response

I decided to call the combined force of these internal influences the faith factor—remembered wellness and the elicitation of the relaxation response. But it became clear that a person's religious convictions or life philosophy enhanced the average effects of the relaxation response in three ways: (1) People who chose an appropriate focus, that which drew upon their deepest philosophic or religious convictions, were more apt to adhere to the elicitation routine, looking forward to it and enjoying it; (2) affirmative beliefs of any kind brought forth remembered wellness, reviving top-down, nerve-cell firing patterns in the brain that were associated with wellness; (3) when present, faith in an eternal or life-transcending force seemed to make the fullest use of remembered wellness because it is a supremely soothing belief, disconnecting unhealthy logic and worries.

I already knew that eliciting the relaxation response could disconnect everyday thoughts and worries, calming people's bodies and minds more quickly and to a degree otherwise unachievable. It appeared that beliefs added to the response transported the mind-body even more dramatically, quieting worries and fears significantly better than the relaxation response alone. And I speculated that religious faith was more influential than other affirmative beliefs.

Does It Matter If You're Devout or in Doubt?

I want to emphasize that the benefits of the faith factor are not the exclusive domain of the devout. People don't have to have a professed belief in God to reap the psychological and physical rewards of the faith factor. With lead investigator Dr. Jared D. Kass, professor at Lesley College Graduate School of Arts and Sciences in Cambridge, Massachusetts, my colleagues and I developed a questionnaire to quantify and describe the spiritual feelings that accompanied the relaxation response, to document their frequency and potential health effects.

Based on the survey responses, we calculated spirituality scores. But because virtually all of our survey respondents reported a "belief in God," this statement could not be used to differentiate people. It was the more amorphous feeling of spirituality that could be linked to better psychological and physical well-being. However, there is one group that does seem more likely to have spiritual encounters. Indeed, women had higher spirituality scores than men, for reasons that we don't yet understand.

Unleash Your Inner Healer

As subjective as remembered wellness is, there are some definitive things that I can say about incorporating healing beliefs and faith into your life. These are some of the principles and practical lessons that I've drawn from my long medical quest for lasting truths. I hope that they prove helpful to you.

Let faith, the ultimate belief, heal you. According to medical research, faith in God is good for us, and this benefit is not exclusive to one denomination or theology. You can believe in God in a quiet, introspective way or declare your convictions out loud to the world—either way, you'll still reap the physiologic rewards.

For many reasons religious activity and churchgoing are also healthy. Religious groups encourage all kinds of health-affirming activities—fellowship and socializing perhaps first among them, but also prayer, volunteerism, familiar rituals, and music. Prayer, in particular, appears to be therapeutic, the specifics of which science will continue to explore.

Trust your instincts more often. People describe the process of finding out what is important to them, of tapping into their beliefs, in very different ways, sometimes calling it soul-searching, mulling it over, listening to one's heart, going inside of one's self, praying, or sleeping on it. Some people act on instincts or common sense; others find that a truth or intuition emerges slowly. But most people know when something feels right. Most people have a kind of internal radar that occasionally calls out to them.

The next time you're faced with a major decision, medical or otherwise, ask yourself, "What feels like the right thing to do?" or "What would I do if the choice were entirely up to me?" I'm not suggesting that you make decisions based on this factor alone, but at least let belief be a player. Honor your convictions and perceptions enough to make them a part of a hearty intellectual argument.

Let your instincts guide you. Follow them up with research. Put your health in good, trustworthy hands. Let your health have time to correct itself. Invest remembered wellness and a reasonable application of self-care, medications, and surgery for maximum health returns.

Practice and apply self-care regularly. Work with your doctor, and with unconventional practitioners if you so choose, to learn self-care habits. I consider self-care anything that an individual can do, independent of doctors or healers, to enhance his health. This includes mind-body reactions such as remembered wellness, the relaxation response, and the faith factor. It also embraces good nutrition, exercise, and other means of stress management.

I use the term *self-care* because it puts the onus on you; it shifts the emphasis from your role as passive patient to active participant—a shift that medicine has not always encouraged. However, I caution against becoming self-absorbed in self-care. Don't become fixated on your health or on the avoidance of aging, illness, or death. Make your daily elicitation of the relaxation response, your jog, or your salad at lunch a no-brainer, which you do not analyze or overthink. Simply delight in the event itself.

It's almost always valuable to seek the assistance of your physician to determine the difference between a condition that will benefit from self-care exclusively and one that requires drugs or procedures to treat. Learning about your body is an evolutionary process. You'll work toward a more independent attitude. Become acquainted with the warning signs of heart attacks, strokes, cancer, and other life-threatening diseases. Over time, you'll develop a sense of what symptoms are important—those that are extreme or don't go away.

How influential can a coordinated contingent of self-care habits be? We honestly don't know, but Dean Ornish, M.D., president and director of the Preventive Medicine Research Institute in Sausalito, California, found that heart disease could not only be relieved but reversed when patients made significant changes in diet, exercise, and stress management. Our two programs will soon be compared in a groundbreaking research project sponsored by the Commonwealth of Massachusetts Group Insurance Commission and the John Hancock Insurance Company. In this comparison patients with heart disease will be divided between our two clinics in hopes that we can gauge the adherence to and results of various self-care components and other treatments.

Beware of people with all the answers. Be careful of any physician, nontraditional healer, spiritual guide, mind-body guru, or any adviser who claims to have all the answers or wants others to think so. Besides love and sex, writers and lecturers today take up few topics with as much evangelistic zeal as health and spirituality. It is no small task shielding these very personal matters from unhealthy speculation and overanalysis, but start with tuning out overly confident or all-knowing mentors and guides. Value your emotions and intuitions the same way your brain does; don't let someone manipulate your wiring for his gain.

Mind-body medicine should remind us of the precious nature of our minds and of the importance of critiquing the messages that we allow to become actualized in our brains and bodies.

Whether or not you believe in God, I believe that we are all wired to crave meaning in life, to assign profound power and sacredness to human experiences, and sometimes even to lend "god" status or "godliness" to humans and human endeavors. Be wary of this tendency, because it may rob spiritual life of its grandeur and of the wonderful transcendent qualities that cannot be accessed entirely by human intellect, and because it makes us very susceptible to human manipulation. Not only is your body a temple, but your mind is an architect, busy transforming the ideas that you feed it. Protect it from those who exploit the power of remembered wellness for personal gain.

Remember that the "nocebo" is equally powerful. Unfortunately, remembered wellness has a flip side. It can have negative side effects, called the nocebo (as opposed to placebo). Our agitated minds may inappropriately trigger the fight-or-flight response in our bodies. Similarly, automatic negative thoughts, bad moods, and compulsive worrying eventually take up physical residence in our bodies. Extreme examples of the nocebo effect include voodoo death, belief-engendered death, mass psychogenic illness, false memories, and "memories" of alien abductions. People who dwell on worst-case scenarios, who exaggerate risks, or who project doubt and undue worry keep the nocebo effect busy in their physiologies. They signal their brains to send help when no physical sickness is present, persuading their bodies to get sick when there is no biological reason why sickness should occur.

Remember that immortality is impossible. While it's healthy to listen to your heart, it's also harmful to deny or duck the truth. No one lives forever. No matter how well-versed you become in mind-body medicine, no matter how far medical progress may be able to set back the clock, death is, like illness and pain, an unfortunate but natural fact of life.

I must sound as if I'm talking in circles, first telling you not to let a diagnosis define you, then warning you not to fall prey to denial. Nonetheless, some lecturers and New Age entrepreneurs imply that all disease is curable and that we can avoid death and aging if we only believe. These salespeople do great harm to people by fostering guilt, and they damage the field of mind-body medicine, which is legitimately trying to establish its findings and change the way Western medicine is practiced. No evidence exists that death can be denied its eventual toll.

Indeed, fear of death can bring out the worst in people, but the realization that death is an inevitable, natural occurrence can also propel healthy, impassioned living.

Living well, exercising and eating appropriately, seeing doctors when you need to but not overrelying on the medical system—these are all proven buffers against disease and illness.

Believe in something good. Even though we do not necessarily need all the pills and procedures that conventional medicine and unconventional medicine give us, these medicinal symbols retain an aura of effectiveness and often appease our desire for action. While we must learn to use medicine more appropriately for the conditions that it can help and wean ourselves from excessive spending on unnecessary therapies, we'll often need some catalysts for belief, even if belief is really the healer.

So remember the vigor from the time when you felt healthiest in your life. Remember the blessing that your mother said to you before you left for school, the smell of incense at church, or the tranquillity that you felt picking up stones from the beach on Cape Cod. Remember the time when the penicillin vanquished your ear infection or the time when the surgeon removed the splinter from deep in your foot and your pain imme-

Pop Your Mind Out of Gear

Stress-management experts recommend that you let your mind slip into idle several times a day so that at least for a few minutes you're not regretting yesterday or fretting about tomorrow. Instead, you're focused on the present moment without feeling compelled to make judgments about your life.

These mental rest stops are important because they can evoke the relaxation response, a physiological state that has been shown to lessen feelings of stress and anxiety. First described by Herbert Benson, M.D., president of the Mind/Body Institute, director of behavioral medicine at Beth Israel Deaconess Medical Center/Harvard Medical School, and author of *Timeless Healing*, the relaxation response reduces muscle tension, lowers heart rate, blood pressure, metabolism, and breathing, and sparks tranquil feelings, says Eileen Stuart, R.N., director of cardiovascular programs at the Mind-Body Institute, a behavioral medicine clinic founded by Dr. Benson at Deaconess Hospital in Boston.

Research also suggests that the relaxation response works in conjunction with spirituality to enhance the body's natural healing power. Proponents say that there are literally dozens of ways to produce the relaxation response, including meditation, yoga, or repetitive prayer. Also, you can use the following bare-bones approach that Dr. Benson says is a distillation of all these disciplines.

First, pick a personally meaningful word or phrase that you can focus on. Sit comfortably and close your eyes. Allow yourself to become aware of your breathing. Each time you inhale, repeat your word or phrase to yourself silently. Thoughts will intrude, but let them drift past. Continue to repeat your word or phrase in a relaxed, passive way for 10 to 20 minutes without trying to make anything happen. If you can, practice this twice a day.

Many people choose a prayer to focus on, Dr. Benson says. So the relaxation response becomes a bridge between medicine and religion. And while adding the power of your faith can make this healing state even more effective, the relaxation response can work without evoking spirituality, he says.

diately ceased. Remember how full-throated you sang in the choir or how long you stayed on the dance floor of a nightclub. Remember the doctor who really cared about you or the chaplain who prayed with you in the hospital. Remember the way you felt when you made love to your spouse, and the way you felt when your daughter or son was born.

Then let go and believe. You've read all about your physiology, and you've surrounded yourself with good caregivers who help you take a moderate, balanced approach to your health and health care. Now it's time to enjoy your endowment, this wiring for faith that makes the power of remembered wellness so enduring.

Believe in something good if you can. Or even better, believe in something better than anything you can fathom. Because for us mortals, this is very profound medicine.

Credits

Portions of Why Use Herbs? on page 3, portions of The Green Grocery on page 27, and portions of Herbal Safeguards on page 45 were adapted from *Nature's Cures*. Copyright © 1996 by Michael Castleman. Reprinted by permission.

Portions of Why Use Herbs? on page 3, portions of The Green Grocery on page 27, Teas and Tinctures on page 30, portions of Herbal Safeguards on page 45, and the "Herbal Solution" box for Stress on page 223 were adapted from *Herbs for Health and Healing*. Copyright © 1996 by Kathi Keville. Reprinted by permission.

What the Neanderthals Knew on page 11 was adapted from *The Healing Herbs*. Copyright © 1991 by Michael Castleman. Reprinted by permission.

Portions of The Healthy Harvest on page 22; portions of Herbal Safeguards on page 45; the "Herbal Solution" for the following chapters: Allergies on page 126, Arthritis on page 132, Back Pain on page 138, Cholesterol on page 145, Colds and Flu on page 148, Heart Disease on page 170, High Blood Pressure on page 181, Natural Weight Control on page 198, Osteoporosis on page 205, Skin Problems on page 213, and Sleep Deprivation on page 218; and portions of the "Herbal Solution" boxes for Digestive Ailments on page 154 and Headaches and Migraines on page 166 were adapted from *The Green Pharmacy*. Copyright © 1997 by James A. Duke, Ph.D. Reprinted by permission.

The recipes for Pear and Ginger Breakfast Muffins on page 250, Sage and Egg Omelet on page 251, Whole-Wheat Spaghetti with Sage on page 253, Broccoli and Potatoes with Dill on page 254, Swordfish with Fennel on page 256, Peppermint Blend Tea on page 256, and Calendula Egg Substitute on page 258 were adapted from *The Good Herb* by Judith Benn Hurley. Copyright © 1995 by Judith Benn Hurley. Reprinted by permission of William Morrow & Company, Inc.

One Week of Natural Healing on page 263 was adapted from *Eight Weeks to Optimum Health* by Andrew Weil, M.D. Copyright © 1997 by Andrew Weil, M.D. Reprinted by permission of Alfred A. Knopf, Inc.

The Wellness within Us on page 287 was adapted with permission of Scribner, a division of Simon & Schuster, from *Timeless Healing: The Power and Biology of Belief* by Herbert Benson, M.D., with Marge Stark. Copyright © 1996 by Herbert Benson, M.D.

Index

Ginkgolic acid, 56
Ginkgolides, 55
Ginseng, **84**, *84*
  buying, 162
  Siberian, 55, 162
  for treating fatigue, 162
Ginsenoside, 162
Glycerin, 33, 35
Glycerine soaps, 213
Glycerites, 33–34, 41
Glycolic acid, 214
Glycosides, 55
Goldenseal, 24, **85**, *85*
Good Herb, The, 249
Good News about High Blood Pressure, 178,
  179, 183
Green Pharmacy, The, 4, 22, 46, 47, 126, 132,
  138, 145, 148, 167, 170, 181, 198,
  205, 213, 218
Gum disease, preventing, 5

H

Hair rinse, vinegars as, 36
Hamamelis virginiana. See Witch hazel
Hamstring stretch for treating back pain,
  136–37, *137*
Hawthorn, **86**, *86*
  for treating high blood pressure, 181
Hay fever, 124–25, 126
HDL. *See* High-density lipoprotein
Headache, **164–69**
  from headphones, 165
  migraine, 4, 164–69
  treating, with
    acetaminophen, 163
    aspirin, 163
    basil, 23
    breathing, deep, 167
    caffeine, 165
    cayenne, 168
    evening primrose, 167
    feverfew, 4, 166–67
    homeopathic remedies, 168
    ice, 164–65
    imagery, 164
    light, 164
    low-fat diet, 165–66
    magnesium, 168
    massage, 169
    nonsteroidal anti-inflammatory drugs,
    163
    nux vomica, 168

    sanguinaria, 168
    sinus irrigation, 168–69
    willow, 167
Headache Help, 164
Health and Healing, 154
Healthy Homestyle Cooking, 146
Heart attack
  preventing, with
    aspirin, 49, 171
    exercise, 174
    thyme, 24
    willow, 4, 49
    wintergreen oil, 49
  sexual activity and, 174
Heartburn, 154–55
Heart disease, **169–75**. *See also* Heart attack
  body mass index and, 172–73
  cholesterol levels and, 175
  preventing, with
    lower sodium intake, 175
    low-fat diet, 174–75
    pigweed, 170–71
    weight loss, 171
  smoking and, 185
  treating, with
    cayenne, 170
    garlic, 170
    ginger, 170
    onions, 170
Hemorrhoids, 157
Hemorrhoids, treating, 157–58
Herb flowers in salads, 255
Herb(s). *See also specific types*
  blends of, 249, 255
  growing and harvesting, **22–25**, 28
    outdoors, **24–25**
    on windowsill, **23–24**
  interactions, 48
  medicinal uses, **3–22**
    animal behavior and, 11–12
    Ayurvedic, 4, 14–15
    Chinese, 10–11, 13–14
    Eclectics and, 20
    Egyptian, 15–16
    European, 16–17
    holistic practice and, 6–7
    homemade products, 39–40
    Native American, 18–19
    regulation of, 5–6, 27–29
    renaissance of, 21–22
  microwaving, 255
  pairing, in cooking, 257
  preparation of
    for external use, 36–40

Y

Z